HARVEY WALDEN'S
NO EXCUSES!
FITNESS WORKOUT

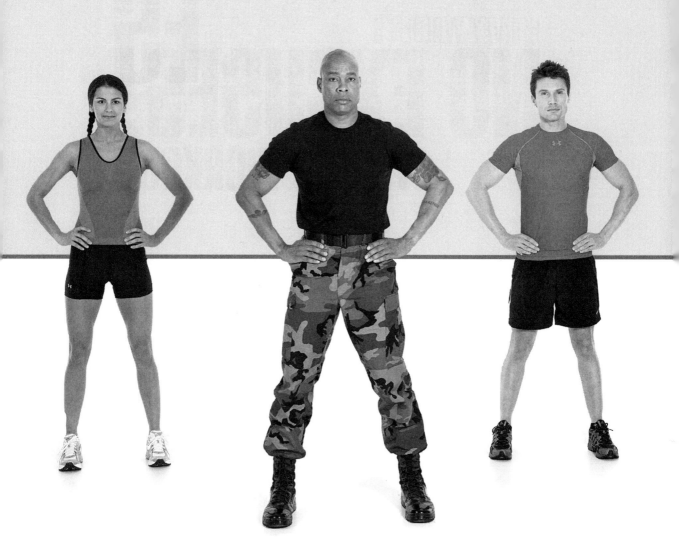

HARVEY WALDEN'S
NO EXCUSES!
FITNESS WORKOUT

HARVEY WALDEN IV

RODALE

© 2007 by Harvey Walden IV

Rodale books may be purchased for business or promotional use or for special sales. For information, please write to:

Special Markets Department, Rodale Inc., 733 Third Avenue, New York, NY 10017

Printed in the United States of America

Rodale Inc. makes every effort to use acid-free ♾, recycled paper ♲.

Book design by Joanna Williams

Photographs by Mitch Mandel/Rodale Images
Photo on page xii by Sheila Lieske

Library of Congress Cataloging-in-Publication Data

Walden, Harvey.
    Harvey Walden's no excuses! fitness workout / Harvey Walden IV.
        p.   cm.
    Includes index.
    ISBN-13 978–1–59486–746–0 hardcover
    ISBN-10 1–59486–746–1 hardcover
    1. Physical fitness. 2. Exercise. I. Title. II. Title: No excuses! fitness workout.
  GV481.W15 2007
  613.7—dc22   2007032303

Distributed to the trade by Holtzbrinck Publishers

2   4   6   8   10   9   7   5   3   1   hardcover

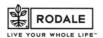

LIVE YOUR WHOLE LIFE™

We inspire and enable people to improve their lives and the world around them

For more of our products visit **rodalestore.com** or call 800-848-4735

To my family and friends who have stood by and supported me in all I do.

To my favorite and only son and daughter Harvey V and Tiyauna, who give me more joy and strength than they will ever know.

To my marines and the Corps who give and sacrifice so much every day without hesitation. OOH RAH and Semper Fidelis!

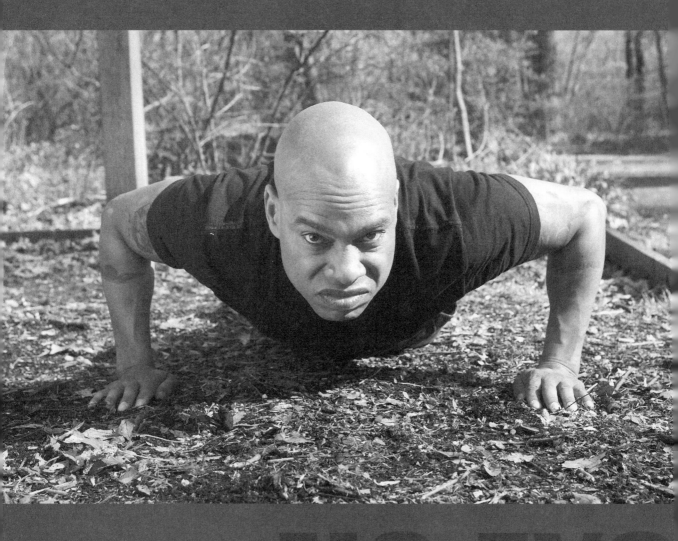

NO EXC

contents

DIG DEEP!

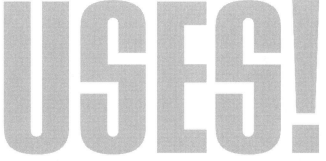

USES!

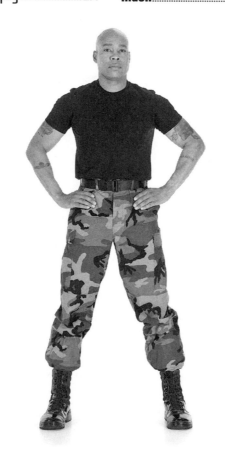

introduction
Take Control of Your Life

What I've gotten from loads of people, whether it has been from people who approach me in public or even at the exercise clinics I host, is: "When are you going to do a workout for the real people who are intimidated by gyms and working out?"

It's a good question and it's so very true: Most overweight people have gym phobias. They hate going out in public places because of the stares they receive from other people.

When I do my exercise clinics, most of the overweight people who attend don't go back to the gym afterward. But they do start walking on a daily basis and watching what they eat. It lasts for a little while, until the motivation they received at the clinic wears off.

I've seen it happen time and again.

I know that people want to lose weight. I see how they enjoy the exercise clinics.

But if you don't have access to an exercise clinic, what do you do?

You start by picking up this book.

Since most people would rather sit at home and watch television, snacking and staying up late, than exercise, I have designed a program that you can do right in your own home.

It will get you fit and give you the confidence to hit the gym, go out in public feeling great about yourself, and have the self-esteem you want and deserve.

It's a quick and healthy way to get up off the couch, out of your comfort zone, and into the fight against fat. My workout is made up of a series of exercises that you can perform even while you are watching your favorite 30-minute TV show. I call it Harvey Walden's No Excuses! Fitness Workout and I mean it. **NO excuses**.

For the first six weeks or so, the workout may look a bit strange to you, but trust me on this and hang in there. It's a series of exercises designed to get your heart rate up, as well as a total body workout that will tone muscle and burn calories, helping you to get the body you want.

Try it and you will be doggone shocked at your weight loss. I guarantee it.

Think of shedding those unwanted pounds like making money. Once we make that money, it goes in the bank and we move on to something else and make more money to get stronger and better. With this program, you'll be laughing all the way to the bank.

Most people need to move around and watch what they eat to lose weight. So this 30-minute workout is designed to maximize movement as well as blast you out of your comfort zone. It's important to change your workout every four to six weeks to keep the body guessing and produce results. If I go to the gym every day and my body gets used to the same exercises and I get into that comfort zone of just plodding along, I won't see any improvements.

For marines, I have to maintain their interest and keep them on their toes, while still developing their muscle memory. When you change your routine and intensity every so often, you make some money and come out of your comfort zone.

After completing each workout, you will have burned loads of calories, and you'll feel good about what you have accomplished.

I think it is best to do your workout first thing in the morning. Maybe you want to do it while watching the morning news, weather, and traffic report. Getting that workout done early will set you up for a productive day and leave you *no excuses* about not having time later or feeling too tired. You also have the option of getting another workout in after work! There you go, now you're kickin' it.

If you do the workout four times a week, in a few weeks' time you'll see the fat falling off and you'll have built up your self-esteem and confidence enough to get into the gym and rock and roll. You'll also learn different variations that will increase the intensity and up the tempo of the workouts.

Believe it or not, I do this workout in my hotel room when I am on the road, have just finished filming, and have some time before a dinner meeting.

I've used the same workout with the celebs at fit camps as with my marines. The key to this is to keep everybody moving, so I take them out to a park and have them form a big circle with laminated cards for each exercise that they perform in a circuit. I have them run around the circle after completing each exercise and before transitioning into the next one.

For you at home, I've included marching on the spot between exercises to achieve that same effect—keeping that heart pumping. This book makes it so easy for you to work out anywhere that you now have **NO excuses.**

The workout has three stages: a Beginner Stage, Intermediate Stage, and Advanced Stage. I also call these stages the Get Off Your Butt Stage, Now You Are in the Fight Stage and Ooh Rah You Are a Stud or Studette Stage. Where you see me use **1st, 2nd,** and **3rd gear,** that tells you how fast you should be exercising, just as if you are driving a car and changing gears.

All you need is this book, a way to keep time (more on this later), and some heart. So let's get started and make some money.

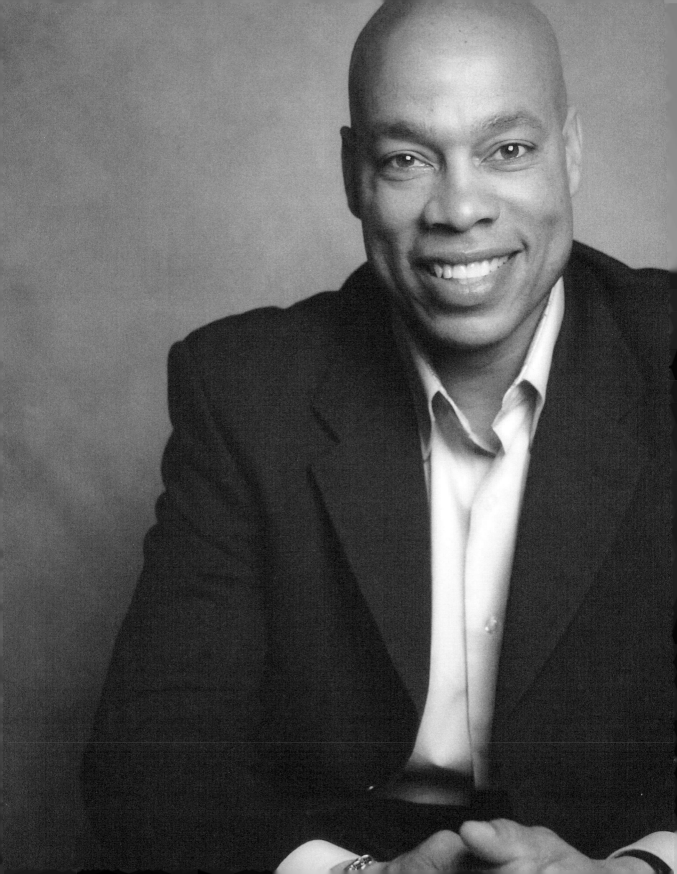

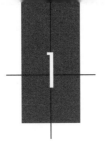

HARVEY WALDEN IV

For as long as I can remember, I'd always wanted to join the army. I was a John Wayne fan, and when I was 13 and saw his movie *The Green Berets,* I knew right away that was where I wanted to be. The discipline he had, he was so cool, strong in his whole character—it impressed me. I thought, *That's for me.*

I've always been an adventurous type of guy, so when I was 16 I set up an appointment with an army recruiter one day after football practice.

My school was on the South Side of Chicago, so just like that, tired, hungry, and sweaty, I went all the way across town to meet this knucklehead, and I get there and he's not there. But I hear something popping! There was a kitchen next to the office, and there was Jiffy Pop cooking.

It was 6:30 and there was no one around. I was hungry and ready for dinner, so I started to eat that popcorn.

So there I am, eating the popcorn, when a big marine comes in. And he starts yelling at me, and he says: "Who do you think you are?"

I said: "I came here to meet the army recruiter and I was hungry."

"So what did the recruiter offer you?" the marine asked.

"He told me I could become a Green Beret."

I was really thinking we were going to have a fight, when he said: "Hey, since you stole my popcorn you gotta come listen to me and hear what the Marine Corps can offer you."

The marine's name was Charlie Childress and he took me under his wing and befriended me, and that was the beginning of a good friendship between us. Joining the marines became my dream.

The other army guy I was supposed to meet never did show up. And as for me, I never looked back.

When I turned 17 I called Charlie up and said: "Hey, look, it's time to see if my dad will sign for me to join the Marine Corps."

Dad didn't want to do it. He wanted me to go to college and become a lawyer. But he did eventually sign the papers.

I did not waste any time—I was out of there like a SCUD missile. I didn't want anything to destroy my goal, and I could see my Chicago friends that summer going to jail, getting shot, getting beaten up. Me, I knew I was leaving Chicago and never coming back.

Boot camp was hell. I was arrogant, cocky, oh man, there was a lot to beat out of me. But they did it. Boot camp is about breaking you down and then building you up again. Into a marine.

These days I'm a drill instructor, I understand the process. When I was 18, though, they had to tear me down and read me my rights a few times before I got the message.

But even then, I showed good leadership—I was good at getting people to do what they didn't want to do and making them love it.

That was probably because I'd had to step up to the plate at home when I was 8 and my parents divorced. My dad was out at school or work all the time, so I was the one taking care of my baby brother, Milton—cleaning, cooking, keeping hold of him.

Today Milton says that I helped him be the person he is now—independent, responsible—and that I've given him the drive to get ahead.

I guess I learned that drive from martial arts which I've been doing from the year dot. Even when I was 4 or 5 years old, I was getting my ass kicked by the big guys. I got my first black belt when I was 6 years old.

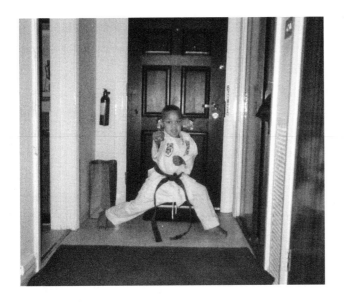

When I'm asked how I motivate people to do some of the things they do, I don't have an easy answer. I can't put it in a bottle. I just know I've been doing it for years. When people struggle with a challenge or exercise course, I tell them to dig deep, find the chi, kick it in the ass, and win the battle.

It's how I've done it with all the marines I've trained.

That's how I grew up knowing how to tap into chi energy. To me, chi energy is the life force that flows through your body. Eastern philosophies have different ways of accessing chi—through acupuncture, martial arts like tai chi, and meditation. Our chi energy is a part of who we are. As a little kid learning martial arts, I heard a lot about chi. Hell, I was so small, I didn't even know what it really was—but I could tell when I was centered and I could feel it flowing. To me, it means finding my inner strength and dropping into my energy reserves to take control of the situation and conquer it.

What I know is that when you think about something being hard, you've already lost the battle. So what I try to do is take that negative energy and rechannel it and put it into something positive.

Everyone needs a motivator, something you can focus on in your mind when you're in trouble, something that makes you happy. Even I have "bad hair" days when I've got to get myself back into the fight. Most of the time my motivators are things like watching my son play football or my daughter play basketball, because she's captain of the basketball team. That's what makes me happier than anything else—my children are my own personal motivators.

In martial arts you learn that if someone pushes you down you've got to know how to roll, how to fall, and how to absorb the blow. You've got to give in so that you can come back up and kick some ass.

That's a good lesson for life too.

So the trick is to find your chi: Relax, breathe easy, believe you can do it.

Roll with the punches—and then come back up.

And you already know: The good things in life don't come easy. When you put in the hard work and make

say: How can I lose 50 pounds in two weeks? I think, *Hell, are you smoking crack? Give me a break.*

You've got to be smart about it. Take small steps, set a long-term goal, but make it realistic. One or two pounds of weight loss a week is enough. We give the celebs on the TV show a little bit more than that to do, because they're in a more controlled environment. But if you're working through this book at home, one or two pounds a week is enough.

It's enough because that's what works. If you set those stepping-stones, then you see that long-term goal that's getting chopped away bit by bit, and

So the trick is to find your chi; Relax, breathe easy, believe you can do it.

sacrifices, and believe me, if you bust your butt, you appreciate what you've achieved later. Don't think it's always going to be red roses. Hell, if it was easy, you'd be a waste of sperm.

It's so doggone easy to take the path of least resistance. It burns me out. People come up to me all the time and

that's all the motivation you need right there, to keep on going toward your aim.

Set up a support system to help you. There are many evil people out there in the world, so surround yourself with good people while you're learning to work out. These people also help you to come back up after you've been knocked down.

My sounding board is the marines. For more than 20 years I've been putting those boots on. You can't replace the camaraderie. It's the most selfless, committed breed you can shake a stick at.

We instill that in marines at boot camp. As drill instructors, we live and eat the marines. That's our life—to be the epitome of what a marine should be, to pass it on. We strip those kids of their identities and we teach them the core values: honor, commitment as a marine, and courage.

When you see those kids first coming off that bus, and then three months later they've got that last day in front of them, and you congratulate them and tell them they've made it, they're marines, and they give you that "Aye, sir!" you get chills up your spine and you think: *That's my boys.*

Over that three-month period, they all become fit. For me, it's a way of life. I've always exercised; it's part of who I am. While it will take some time for you to lose weight and to get fit, if you make working out a part of your life, it will come naturally. And it pays off big

time. I know a lot of people my age who look a whole lot older. If you're fit, you're healthier, you're mentally stronger. You can take all the memory-enhancing pills you want to, but stay physically healthy and you'll have memories that will last.

Being fit makes you stronger emotionally as well. It means you can deal better with what life throws at you. And that's important. When I look back at the people I grew up with, I don't even recognize some of them now. An unhealthy life, eating fried chicken and never moving, man, it clogs up your arteries, makes you pile on the pounds, look a lot older, and you've got a shorter life ahead of you. There's nothing wrong with a little social drinking, and cognac and red wine are good for you. But don't drink too much.

I found out about healthy eating a long time ago, when I was 9 or 10, because one day I got very sick. I'd snuck to a burger joint a block from the school and bought a cheeseburger. I felt so bad once I was back at school that they thought I was going to throw up, and they sent me home.

That day my dad found me on the kitchen floor.

I never ate a cheeseburger again. For a long time after that, all I cooked was spaghetti and steamed vegetables. My little brother hated it, but it did us both good in the end.

I got into doing the television show *Celebrity Fit Club* by accident. I was 32 and stationed in London with a security force company, with offices in Grosvenor Square and Eastcote, not too far from West Ruislip. We were responsible for the security of the commander in chief of Naval forces in Europe, and I had a tough schedule and a lot to do, so I was in the gym at 5:00 a.m. every day and didn't go to bed until midnight.

I've always liked England—its history, its culture. It became home to me. I spent almost five years there—from 1998 to 2002. The camaraderie I had in the Marine Corps, I saw in England everywhere. The English football team where I played, the London Mets—man, those guys had my back. The London Mets are the best guys you could hope for in the world.

One day we heard that the Granada production company was interviewing trainers for a show called *Fat Club* that would air in the United Kingdom on ITV. I'd always been a personal trainer and I'm not sure if they saw me at the YMCA or what, but someone from Granada called the U.S. Embassy looking for me.

As it happened I was in Washington, D.C., for a conference at the time, and Colonel Stemley, the defense attaché at the U.S. Embassy in London, called me and said: "Hey, these producers have been here looking for you for some freakin' TV show and I think you should do it."

I said no, being the marine I was, but Lee Servis, the producer of *Fat Club*, was very persistent. He asked me to have lunch with him. We met and had a pint and Lee had a camera with him. Back then, I didn't realize I was having a screen test right there in the pub. That was to see how I looked on camera. In the end, I agreed to take part.

Fat Club was the first show I did. It was based in London. We had everyday people and they were extremely overweight. I was under the impression that I was helping people lose weight, but had no idea that they would all be close to 300 pounds—and some so big we had to use a post-office scale to weigh them.

The very first day we filmed, I was worried how I was going to get them to lose weight because I had never trained people with so much weight to lose. When they walked in through that door I admit it, I wanted to jump straight up and get out of there.

At the break I said to Lee, "What are y'all expecting me to do with these people?" But Lee was so smooth, he said: "Train them—you can do it." He knew I wouldn't quit.

It was a big challenge for them and for me. They were very, very heavy people and they had never been near a gym.

So I started by putting them in a cold pool.

At 5:00 a.m. the first day of the show, I came downstairs and turned off the heat. By the time the cameras were rolling an hour later it was real icy, and man, were they cold. I had them swim laps and after about 15 laps asked them how they felt. They were mad. In fact, one girl wanted to kick my freaking ass; then they all got out of the water and they *all* wanted to kick my ass.

But I said: "I know you're feeling angry, but do you see why I did that? You've achieved something, something physical, and now you've got a gauge. Now you can see that exercise is easy. You just force yourself out of your comfort zone and do it. You didn't want to get up this early and you didn't want to swim in cold water, but you accomplished it. We got the hard part out of the way first, so now let's exercise and you'll see that you can do that too."

I asked them how they would compare swimming in a cold pool to just going for a walk. Which of the two would they rather do? Which would be easier to accomplish if I wasn't here to make them jump in the pool? They all said they would rather go for an early-morning walk.

Not many people will get up in the early morning to go for a swim in a cold pool. They didn't like it, but hell, shit happens. I caught a lot of flak about that on the first day, but the method behind my madness was that these people were extremely overweight and they did not want to exercise at all. My

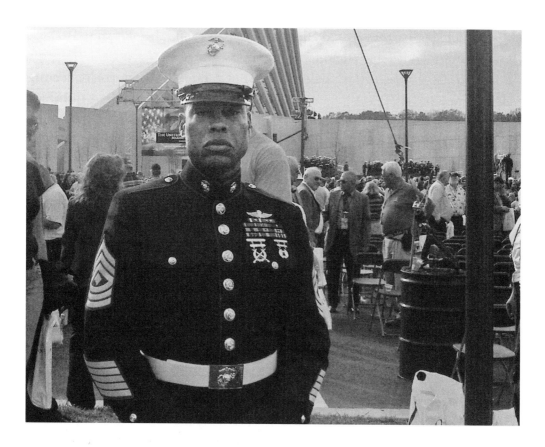

goal was for them to get in the cold pool, knowing they were going to complain and whine. I had to show them something they COULD do.

And it worked. It worked very well. In fact, Tony, one of the guys from that first show, became a very successful personal trainer himself.

So that was me: a full-time marine during the week and a TV fitness trainer on the weekends.

I would work in the Marine Corps in Quantico from Monday to Friday, and every Friday night I'd fly from Washington to London, arriving Saturday morning. When I stepped off the plane I was taken straight to the set, where I'd film all that day and Sunday morning, and then catch a plane back to D.C. That went on from November to March for the first season of *Celebrity Fit Club*.

For five years I worked this way. I moved from London to Washington, DC, in 2002 and from DC to Fort Knox, Kentucky, in 2005. There I'd get to the gym at about 6:00 a.m., finishing work at about 18.00 hours (6:00 p.m.). Even during my breaks or on the airplane, I'd work or catch up on e-mails. Every week I would answer questions for my Ask Harvey Web site here in the States, and for articles for magazines and papers in London.

Nobody can top me at time management. You need those skills if you're going to accomplish your goals. Anyone can learn them, it'll cost you nothing and it will change your life. If you're sitting around doing nothing, you're wasting time. And time is precious—you don't get too much of it. I didn't get any time off.

To fit in two full-on careers and run them side by side, I had to learn to prioritize. I always make a list the day before, so I can start hitting right away the next day.

I do it while I'm working out in the gym. That's when I go through my mental Rolodex and I think about what's going on for the next day. When I go for a run it's even better: I can get

a whole month planned in my mind. I get back in the locker room and jot down everything I've thought of, and when I get back to my office I write everything down on my calendar.

I could not have accomplished any of this without planning, time management, and energy. That's why you've got to be fit and eat healthily: to be able to reach your goals.

Planning helps you reach your goals successfully because it is only when you plan that you know what your goal really is. Once you've got a lock on that goal, if you don't manage your time well, you fail. You have to get your priorities in order and allocate your time according to your priorities. Figure out what you've got to do and stick to the plan. In order to stick to the plan, you have to have discipline. And to accomplish anything, you have to have energy. Reaching your goals makes you feel better about yourself, and that creates more energy.

At first I was a bit too forceful with the celebs. I learned that I had to be more tactful with them than I had to be with the marines. But by the end of the show many of the celebs became my friends. To this day, I'm still in touch with some people from the early shows.

As a trainer, I deal with women and men in the same way. I'm known for being firm, but I'm also consistent and fair. If the female is taking the easy way out I don't give her an easier time. I'm going to call her on it just the same as I would any man.

How many people want to get dirty and crawl in mud? I say to the celebs: "You say you ain't going to the gym, but look at you, you just crawled in freakin' nasty mud. You never thought you'd do that, did you? Now you can go to the gym as well."

And ropes. No one ever believes they can climb a rope. It's a physical chal-

The good things in life don't come easy, if they did you wouldn't appreciate them. So stop your whining and start making some money!

My aim is always to bring out the best in people. I don't tell them anything they don't know. I don't play mind games with them. I tell them the truth, that's all. And their lives get better. When they come in overweight, they need help—and that's what I'm there for.

So I start with challenges they can accomplish. Even someone very overweight and unfit can do a 30-minute power-walk. I love using mud and rope courses to begin to break down people's resistance to change.

lenge and a great way to get people feeling that sense of accomplishment and pride in what they can do. The rope course down at Bakersfield, I like that one because for every obstacle, every rope, you have to get in the mud. I remember how Chastity Bono, Cher's daughter, hit the wall on the rope and couldn't get any higher. But I climbed up there and talked her through it and she did it. She had a rope burn, and the next day at the weigh-in she pulled her shirt up and said: "I've got a war wound!" She was proud of what she'd done.

Once we get the people moving, we do a complete training program for them for the whole 100 days. I give them a three-tier workout schedule for the first six weeks, of four days a week with lots of different exercises, followed by a fun day—salsa or freakin' tango or a hip-hop dance class, we'll do something that still gets their heart rates up.

Because we can't keep them in a totally controlled environment for the full 100 days, I give them choices. I give them the tools. I tell them how much weight they need to lose—but then it's up to them.

I know it's hard for them. It's a mental challenge to plan, manage their time, and make sure that they have the energy to do it all. They don't want to fail, or embarrass themselves on national TV, and this is one thing they can't hire anyone else to do. Their publicists and drivers and personal assistants can't do it for them. They have to do it for themselves. For some of them, it might be the first time.

And some continue their plan long after they have been on the show. I recently got an e-mail from Wendy Kaufman telling me that she was back on the plan and back in the fight. "The thought of seeing you next to me scares me, so I'm committed again," she wrote.

Just like the celebs on the show, if you're using this book to work out, you need to vary the routines. Follow the three-tier workouts and change every six weeks. That way you stay fresh and you stay in the fight.

Training marines is totally different from working on the shows. On the base, I'm training warriors, guys that have to go in harm's way and provide freedom for the nation. You can't compare that to the celeb life. If you think it is in any way comparable, you're insulting what a marine stands for.

Working as a drill instructor, I have to begin by stripping the new recruit's identity. I don't need someone coming in with bad habits; I'm training a marine to follow orders, be a basic trained marine, build esprit de corps, take on the core values. I never forget that that kid may have to face some tough decisions and still find a way to come back home.

I push the envelope with the marines a lot more than with the celebs. And my platoon has to be the best, so I

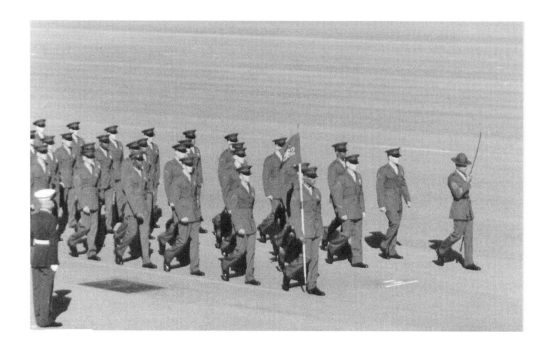

make them do circuit training to get strong bodies, with ten different stations in a circle. I place laminated sheets with instructions at the stations and the marines have to follow them, and I keep them moving.

When I'm training my marines, I know that there is nothing worse than setting out without a plan. They expect you to show them the right way, and you are there to be organized and to teach them to be the same. You're passing the torch. Believe me, they never forget it. At my retirement ceremony in June 2007, every platoon did a little skit about how I trained them. At the end, one marine stood up in front of everyone and said, "Thank you for what you've taught us about leadership—and for being on the watch all my life." Planning, time management, and discipline. That's how you win.

With this book it's the same. Keep moving, just like the marines in training, and vary the exercises, just like the celebs. This way you'll stay fresh and stay in the fight. Follow the instructions and take it one day at a time. That's how you'll win the fight.

I realize that you have a very busy

schedule, but believe me, you can learn to manage your time and you can stop making excuses about why you can't get fit. You are going to dig deep and find the reasons why you can.

Once you're working out, you can find lots of ways to keep moving. Plan trips—go hiking, bike riding, or to the beach. It's something you can do with your family—and then you're helping the next generation get fit too. A good half-hour workout is all it takes to break the cycle of excuse making. A half hour a day that can change your life. That's what this book is for. I guarantee that if you will commit to doing this workout for the first six weeks, the rest will get easier. You'll begin to see results, and it will make you proud of what you've accomplished.

It's your life and you can get control of it. Stand tall, dig deep, and get into the fight!!

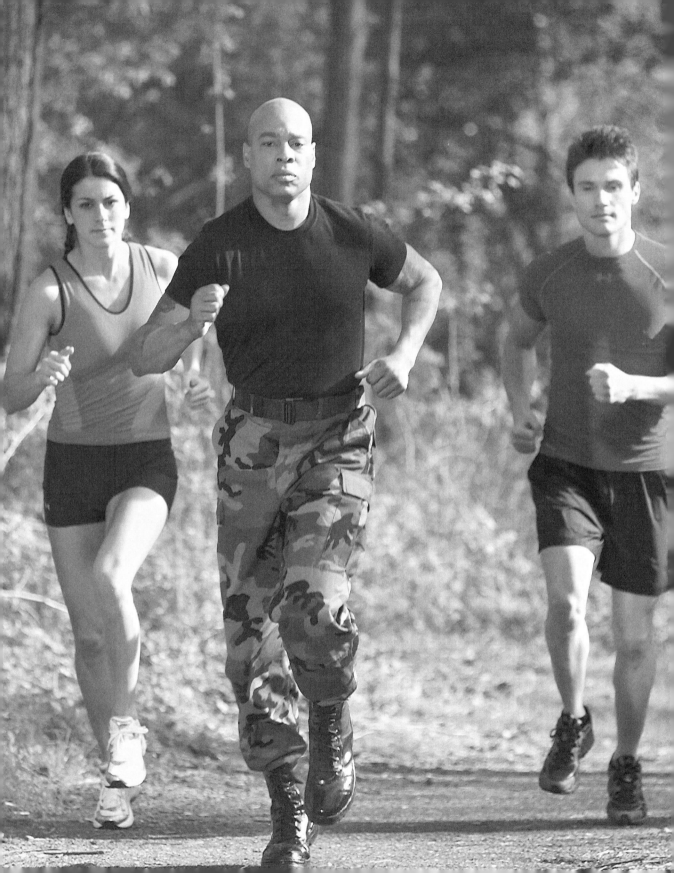

2

WHY BEING FIT IS THE ULTIMATE GOAL!

LOOK, if you decide to get into the fight and stay with it as a lifestyle choice, the benefits are going to be huge.

You are going to live longer and while you are living longer, you're going to feel better, feel stronger, and also be mentally fit for the road ahead.

You know that life is going to throw all kinds of things in your way. That's just the way it is, and if you are prepared and ready for anything, then you are going to cope with it better and come out on top.

Be positive. A positive attitude toward your own body is a real plus in life, because if you ain't gonna look after it, who is?

Most of us know we could be in better shape but we just put it off; say we'll do it tomorrow and tomorrow never comes. People just sit their fat butts on the couch, turn on the TV, and reach for some sugary, salty, snacky, easy food to chew on.

This is not good, and if you want an early out from this life, then that's a good way of helping stack the odds against you. But is that fair to your kids? Your family and friends? Hell no, of course it isn't. They all want you around for as long as possible, so why not give yourself a fighting chance?

Would you walk across the road with your eyes shut when you could open them? You can get into shape and you will enjoy it. That's what the No Excuses! plan is about. It is tough, but I KNOW it works. I have seen it in action and I have witnessed the rewards.

People do need motivations to get them into the zone and keep them there and focused. Even me.

I carry a picture of actress Halle Berry with me in my workout journal wherever I go. It's from a magazine and she's in a boxing ring. It motivates me if I'm slipping because that picture inspires me. It's not a sexual thing, although she is great looking. It's because it shows her in great shape, a great statement of fitness, and the life force just flows out of her, I think. That picture keeps me on the straight and narrow.

Even though I have had physical fit-ness in my life from the age of 4, we all get tempted to be lazy, to eat junk food, and to engage in other behaviors that tear us down. I'm no different.

I can hang out with pals and, while I will mostly take the sensible food option and watch the portion control, I might have too many beers one night or a cognac, which is a treat for me, with one of my friends who keeps me up late on the odd occasion. I'll get up the next day and work extra hard to work it off.

It's okay to fall down once in a while; we're all human. But you need to know that you can grab it back by getting back in line and getting to work the next day.

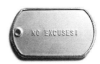

So we know that being in shape makes us feel better about ourselves and life. I tend to believe that it makes life look better on us too, like you make your own luck. The harder you work, the luckier you get.

It seems obvious to me that if you walk into an interview and have a glow from feeling tight and honed and con-fident about your body shape, that message is going to get over to the guy on the other side of the desk.

If you slouch in, belly falling over your belt, butt hanging off the seat, breathing hard because you just had to walk up a small flight of stairs, what's his first thought?

You might be excellent at your job and have a glowing résumé, but more often than not, first impressions count. If there's someone up against you with similar qualifications but who comes across fitter and faster, then they'll probably get the nod.

It's like on *Celebrity Fit Club*, those guys come to us because they want to get the spark back in their lives. They know it will help their career prospects when they show up at an audition and they look like they can handle a heavy schedule.

In showbiz there are so many temptations. Lots to drink, food and more food, late nights, party, party, party. It's okay for a while, maybe, but that stuff's gonna get you, baby. You may as well admit it, but nobody does. They have to fall down first before they learn. Then, if they're lucky, they can get back up again.

We've seen them come crawling in, and I think "Oh my God, we've got some work to do with this one." I can tell if people are fit for the fight pretty much straight off. It's a first impression I get. I've got a sixth sense about it. I suppose that comes from spending my life in and around exercise.

You have to approach people in different ways with different motivations, but generally you can get through to people on different levels. And we have. But our results are pretty good.

Everybody on *Celebrity Fit Club* has to have a thorough physical before we start, so we know what we are up against. We have all the stats, we know the problems and the mountain the celebs must climb.

Most celebrities are used to being mollycoddled, surrounded by people who do everything for them, gofers who say "yes" all the time. And here I am ready to say "no." But I tell 'em why and wherefore and that I'm not just being mean for the fun of it; there is a point and they are going to get my point, like it or lump it.

They WILL get the message.

We had Vincent Pastore, who played Salvatore "Big Pussy" Bonpensiero, on the HBO show *The Sopranos*, and I'm pretty sure it proved to be a blessing for him because he really wasn't in the greatest shape when he arrived.

He'd had heart surgery a year prior and turned 60 with us on the show. He was known as a quitter and has admitted that since, but I wasn't going to let him quit on me. We got along so well, he responded and did himself proud.

One day I had set up a fire hose that the celebrities had to carry up a flight

And after that, I know he felt better about himself and wasn't quite so ready to be a quitter. That man was incredible.

But what it also did was to push the others to achieve their goals. If Vincent could do it, why couldn't they?

Vincent stayed with the program and got himself into better and better shape. Just a year before he'd had life-saving surgery. Now he'd been given a second chance. He was right to fight

We are only here for a short time, so why stack the cards against you and tap out early?

of stairs, and it was proving to be a hard test for them all. But Vincent managed to make it all the way up despite it being a real struggle.

He said later he'd heard me yelling and encouraging him from the top of the stairs and he was determined to make it up there. It was a challenge and he got into the fight and stayed there till he won. I was real proud of him because he was the oldest and had heart issues, but still he got home safely and strongly.

the fight to try to get into better shape and look after his refurbished heart.

That's the point, and it is part of my message that keeping fit and active is for life, not a few months.

Get into good habits and the good habits will get into you and help in every way.

Vincent showed us that it is never too late to start getting fit.

That was also the case with one of my friends from the British version of *Fit Club,* Russell Grant, a well-known astrologer and TV star. He'd also had serious heart problems not too long before participating in the show and was very overweight.

Russell was there to find new life in that body, because he was a very smart guy, with lots of interests and pursuits, but, like everyone, knew his brain was in far better shape than his pudgy body.

He was known as a cuddly, cute guy, short and smiley. But when he got checked out, his statistics were horrifying.

In front of millions watching live on British television he was told that clinically he was in danger of dropping dead at any moment.

Nobody had ever seen such a set of figures.

Poor Russell, who was also in his fifties, gulped heavily, went a little white, and said something like he'd better get on with getting fitter before it was too late . . . too true.

Man, that dude was a walking heart attack waiting to happen.

It kind of shocked all the other celebrities, and at that moment a bond formed between many of them. This inspired Russell too, because so many people cared about him. And that applies to you too. In your tough moments, when you think that you are letting only yourself down, think about all the people who care about you. Stay in the game.

Even so, Russell had some tough moments, and let's understand here, this isn't just about your body, it's about your brain too—kind of mind against flab—and psychologically you have to get fit to fight. He gradually, pound by pound, lost a lot of weight and felt a whole lot better about himself and his chances.

The watching public also helped, by sending in letters and e-mails, urging him to stick with it, go for the targets I set, and lose the weight.

Hopefully a lot of people at home are inspired to get themselves into better shape after seeing what we can achieve with the celebrities. That is one of my motivations for doing the show, to encourage people to get in that fight.

And, as I write this, Russell is very much alive. And he has a new lease on life.

Now let's think about that mental attitude.

I have "bad hair" days. You have "bad hair" days. We all do.

I try to get over mine by going for a long run. I just pound along, mile after mile along tank trails near my base, and I find that it just washes through my brain, clearing my head. When I get back I feel totally refreshed and ready for whatever the day brings.

Of course, I've been running for a lifetime, so it's not for everyone right away.

I will talk in more depth later about getting into running, but, for the moment, just concentrate on moving and how it helps you to clear your mind. Remember that any movement is an improvement over none.

First, I would say to start out with some power-walking. I just love walking, and unless you have some medical condition, everyone can start on the journey back to healthy living by getting off their fat butts and getting a good long walk in. And build up the pace because that really makes a difference.

Think like you are racing to get that train and you can't run, but have to stroll really quickly to make it in time, or you'll be late for work or that important date.

Try it. You won't regret it. Find yourself a safe route through a safe neighborhood or the countryside, maybe where other people are exercising or relaxing. This is supposed to be fun, so breathe in and let go of anything that is stressing you out while you are out and about.

Make it fun. Make it a break for yourself. Take a phone, a music player, a dog, or a friend. Take a break to breathe in the air, take in that spectacular view. Meditate a little. Turn negative energy into positive energy. Put the energy of temptation to work. Sure beats pigging out on candy bars watching daytime soaps.

Movement helps you cope with life in general. We get so many things that come up and smack us in the face, why bring on anything by being a lazy-ass? There are many things we can't control in life, but there are some things that we can influence. Two of those are fitness and healthy eating.

I'm no doctor and I don't pretend or claim to be any kind of a medical expert, but a healthy lifestyle surely can help prevent and/or fight many illnesses. I see it with my own eyes all the time.

On *Celebrity Fit Club* we see so many people with unhealthy lifestyles coming in with signs of type 2 diabetes, which isn't going to be good for their future chances. So we know that from the early physical, and it's all part of what we work on with our food and fitness regimes. At the end of the 100 days, they leave with no signs of the

really proud of them because I hadn't told them what to say. I wouldn't anyway. They have their own minds and can express themselves very well.

Tiyauna, who was then about 14, said she always liked to eat healthily because she knew if she ate trashy foods she just wouldn't be able to run up and down the soccer field or the

You are in control of your life!

disease at all. They, like our friend Russell, literally have a new lease on life.

When I look around the United States and Europe I'm absolutely horrified at how many obese children there are. The obesity rates everywhere are climbing, and that means an earlier death and a pretty unhealthy and often unhappy life on the way to it.

As adults, we can't ignore this situation because it's our fault. We are parents and we should be decent role models for our young. How can we expect them to get on the right track if we lead them from birth down the wrong one?

I took my son and daughter to London four years ago when I was doing some television interviews, and they took part in one major broadcast. I was

basketball court. She said what she puts in her body gives her the energy to compete in her sport.

And my son, Harvey V, who was 10, said he knew that if he sat around all day eating candy, he just wouldn't have the energy to play football.

I think you can lecture kids to death, but if they see you preaching something and not practicing it, they won't give a rat's ass about what you are saying. But I'll guarantee that if they see you doing the right thing and getting results, they will pick up on it and do it for themselves.

I think that's why I have been so successful in the marines; I don't give those kids any bull. I live what I teach. If I didn't, they'd see right through it.

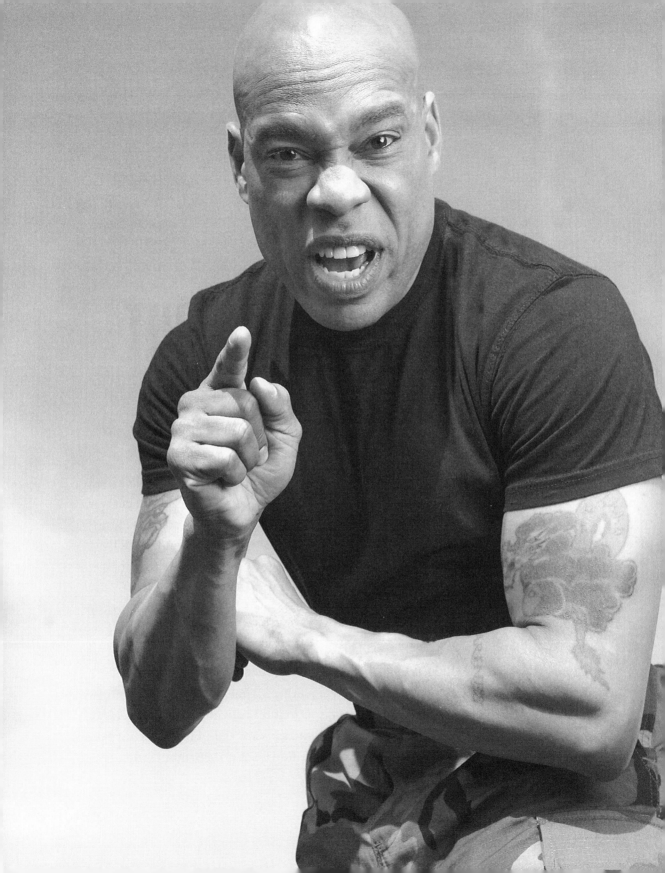

3

PLAN TO WIN— GETTING IN THE FIGHT

By now, you must know that you have to get fired up to get started. Heck, you were motivated enough to buy the book, so you must be interested in getting fit and eating more nutritious and beneficial food.

So that's a really good start. We are getting on the road, my friend. Let's keep getting it hot and make some money. Because your whole life is going to be better for it. What more motivation do you need?

I don't think there's any difference in motivating the rookie recruit in the marines or the new celebrity on *Celebrity Fit Club* or the slob at home on his couch. Everybody can be motivated. You just have to find the thing that turns them on or pisses them off.

Getting mad can motivate you too. Getting somebody fighting mad moves them to action. If I can't find the thing in their life or personality that gets them going, I whup 'em up, get them riled, and turn all that raw power into positive energy, energy to get the job done and feel good because they have achieved something.

In season three of *Celebrity Fit Club* (2006), actress-singer Countess Vaughn was having a really hard time. She broke down during a weigh-in and revealed she was having some trouble back at home because she was going through a painful divorce and couldn't focus on sticking to the right diet and exercising.

She's the only person in the history of the club who actually put on weight—4 pounds. And that upset her.

But despite all her problems, Countess did have one thing that pushed her and motivated her. That was my job. That's what I do. I spot that thing.

So one day when she was in camp and the routine involved climbing a rope to ring a bell, she was on the verge of quitting halfway up.

So Kelly LeBrock and I climbed up there and got into the moment and I told her: "Hey, look, relax, breathe easy. You can do this. It's mind over matter— if you don't mind, it doesn't matter.

"Now ring that doggone bell for your baby boy. Hey, that bell, that's him. That's what he wants you to do. He wants you to succeed. Do it for him if you don't want to do it for yourself. Don't quit on him now."

And hand over hand, she clawed her way up that rope and rang that bell and started crying and came down and gave me a big hug. Man, was she happy.

I knew the one thing she loved to death in life was her son, and that was the motivation she needed to get the hell up that rope and do her job.

Maybe when things get tough for you, think of your children or parents or girlfriend or boyfriend. Do it for them. They want you to succeed. Think how good you'll feel if you ring that personal bell of yours.

You want to tell them you did it; you want to tell them how much weight you've lost or how far you've run or how you've power-walked four miles faster than ever before.

You can be a winner. You can achieve your goals. You've just got to engage your brain and sign up for the plan and go for it.

I had a little trouble getting that message across to rapper Da Brat in season five (2007). We had a big fight right at the beginning, but now we are good friends and text each other every so often to see how we are doing.

I like to keep in touch with the *Celebrity Fit Club* members. They know if they start to drift and need a talk, they only have to call and we can sort something out. So Da Brat is a pal now, and I like the lady a lot. She even calls me "mate," which is a term like "buddy" that I picked up while I was living in England, and she learned it from me. It sounds funny coming from a gangsta rapper.

But it wasn't always like that. In fact, it looked like I was going to be one of her biggest enemies, and that isn't a great position to be in.

Right from the start she was ready to quit. She was going to just up and walk off the set. And she's the kind of girl who does what she says.

She doesn't so much threaten as promise, if you know what I mean.

But on the first day, she turned up and arrived with all this attitude, trying to tell me how it was done. I had to gently tell her I was in charge, not her, and it got really ugly. We were in each other's faces having a real war.

Well the way is MY way in the club; otherwise, those guys are just going to

If you don't mind it won't matter. Stop whining and make some money. Work it out!

take the rip and never get fit. They might think it's a joke, but I tell them in no uncertain way that it's not.

Da Brat was like many of the others who were used to getting their own way. She was surrounded by people who waited on her hand and foot, asskissers, and I don't do that. No way, man. She tells everybody what to do and expects that of everyone. Well, that's not me either.

She met her match in me, and even though she's a girl and I don't disrespect women in any way, shape, or form, I had to let her hear my side of the argument, which is the right side.

It's my job to get these folks in line and get them fit and help them find their aim in order to hit the targets we set for them, which is all in their best interests.

Da Brat isn't very tall and she weighed in at 172 pounds, so there was plenty of work to do.

For the entire first weekend she was of me. Once she realized I was on her side and that I was not her enemy, she saw that together we could win the battle.

When I first started doing the show about five years ago, I thought it would be quite easy to work with people who had volunteered to come on *Celebrity Fit Club* and work on their weight.

But so many of them get the gig and then realize it's a whole lot of hard work and they really just want to con-

You can be a winner. You can achieve your goals. You've just got to engage your brain and sign up for the plan and go for it!

at war with me. I wasn't backing off. It's like so many people who come in there. They want to lose weight, but they want to do it on their terms. But I kept her at it and she came around and really did a good job. Again, I had been forced to find a point at which she was motivated.

With Da Brat it was that anger that I used to turn into a positive energy to throw at her workouts and diet instead tinue in their bad old ways. Sound like anybody you know?

Motivation can strike in many ways. In season four (2006), former *Baywatch* star and *Playboy* Playmate Erika Eleniak wanted to get back in shape to relaunch her career after having a baby daughter.

But, without a doubt, she was the best we ever had on the show. She had her target clearly in sight and she

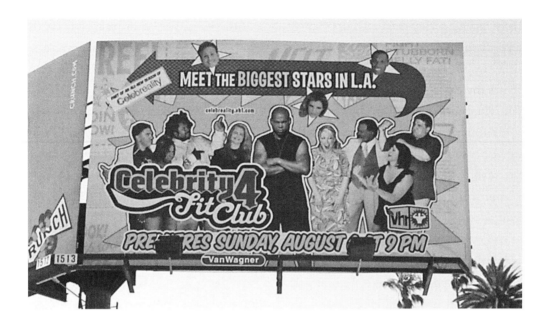

aimed right for it. You've got to have a target.

I was getting reports back from trainers saying, "This girl is a beast; whatever we throw at her she just nails."

In the fit camp I fixed up a mini-triathlon and she just kicked ass in it. So when she was up on the scales I said, "Damn, Erika, what else can I give you to do? Everything we set, you just eat it up." She said: "Whatever you've got, bring it on and I'll do it."

I wanted to find something really exciting because I didn't want her to lose that force that was driving her to achieve all these goals. It's something I believe in big time: making exercises interesting and also at the same time keeping the contestants, and marines for that matter, guessing about what is coming next.

I don't want people to yawn and say: "It's an easy one next," or "Oh, oh, it's that real bitch up next, I'll save some energy."

So what I did through VH1 connections with the Ultimate Fighting Championship and Chuck Liddell, the then champ, was to get a training session with those guys, and believe me, it doesn't get any tougher than that.

They are beasts—nice guys away from the octagon, but fitness freaks who don't know when to stop.

Erika was a Chuck fan, so she was delighted and, of course, she got through the session with ease.

So my advice to you is to take a good look at yourself in the mirror. Think about what motivates you and what you will need to get you on your journey and to keep you there. Plan it out. There'll be a few roadblocks along the way, but we all get those. I do allow for a few "cheat" days when you can go off the rails for a short time. Not too many and not too often. Just enough to have a balance and allow a little naughtiness into your life. Like a couple of beers or a few fries or a little cognac . . .

My No Excuses! plan has been designed over several years. It will take you step-by-step through the three stages to a level of fitness that will be a reward in itself because well before reaching the highest level you will be feeling better about yourself and life in general.

But what I also want you to do is to create a diary, so you can plan your week ahead. I think it is vital to have the week targeted.

I want you to do my workout four times a week. So set your days and the time you can do it, maybe leaving a rest day in between, depending on work and social commitments.

But remember this is the NO EXCUSES! plan. So I will not listen to anyone saying they were at a convention somewhere and couldn't do it. You didn't just find out today that you had to go to that convention. You can fit in half an hour any day. Anywhere. I know YOU can because I do.

So perhaps you can start your week on a Monday. Rest on Tuesday. Work out on Wednesday. Rest on Thursday. Work out on Friday and Sunday. But have a night out with the boys (or girls) on Saturday. Take it easy, though. Don't blow all your hard work on one night.

Use any schedule that will suit you, keeping in mind that you are more likely to hit your target if you take aim, meaning plan the week ahead with as much information as you

PLANNING AND PREP

Use this page as a sample to create your own weekly commitment page.

PROMISE YOURSELF: "I will work out 4 times a week for 30 minutes."

To be successful:

- Plan your workout times for the full week ahead. Make an appointment with yourself four days a week. Remember to leave time after your 30-minute workout to rest and take a shower.

- Plan at least one day of shopping so that you will have all the food you need on hand when you are ready to eat. Plan at least one hour for each shopping trip so that you are sure to get all of the right foods and you won't have to rush your choices.

- Make an appointment with yourself to create your shopping list.

- Schedule time for food preparation. Some people like to prep all their food a couple of times a week and some like to prepare every meal fresh. It is up to you but make sure you plan to have the right food available.

- Schedule your weigh-in once a week. It is best to weigh in on the same day, at the same time, and with the same amount of clothing to get an accurate reading on your weight loss.

Sunday	Monday	Tuesday	Wednesday	Thursday	Friday	Saturday
	1 *weigh-in* *6 am —exercise*	2	3 *7 pm—spin class*	4	5 *6 am—exercise*	6 *7 am—meet* *Jane for walk*
7 *grocery* *shopping*	8 *weigh-in* *6 am —exercise*	9	10 *7 pm—spin class*	11 *6 am—exercise*	12 *7:30 Dr. appt.* *walk after work*	13
14 *6 am—exercise*	15 *weigh-in* *6 am —exercise*	16	17 *7 pm—spin class*	18	19	20 *7 am—meet* *Jane for walk*
21 *grocery* *shopping*	22 *weigh-in* *6 am —exercise*	23 *6 am—exercise*	24 *7 pm—spin class*	25 *6 am—exercise* *Jenna's science* *project*	26	27
28	29 *weigh-in* *6 am —exercise*	30 *walk after work*				

have about how the week is going to lay out. That way, you will be able to maneuver around the surprises, and you can respond and reschedule to get all your workouts in. Be realistic about it and plan it like you do other appointments. And leave enough time to shower and rest up for a few minutes.

My workout can be done morning, noon, or night and even in front of the TV while you are watching your favorite show. You CAN do both at once. It's just a question of training yourself to combine the activities.

So I want to see that personal fit club diary being organized on paper, PDA, cell phone, whatever, and I also want you to write down what mood you are in when you start the exercise and what mood you are in when you finish. You'll be surprised.

Have some realistic targets too. Say you want to lose one pound in the first week. If you lose more you will be delighted with yourself. But don't overdo it. To lose too much weight too quickly is as bad as putting weight on. So be reasonable with yourself.

Your doctor can help you plan out how much weight to lose week by week. You certainly must get a full checkup before embarking on this course and we will talk in more depth about that in later pages.

Weigh yourself regularly, but not too regularly. We don't want to introduce any negative elements that can play tricks on your mind, such as putting on the odd pound for some reason. We all fluctuate a little for natural reasons. I suggest weighing once a week at the same time each week and with similar clothing on.

While you are planning your exercise days, I also want you to plan what you are going to eat. Do the shopping. It's all part of the preparation and the new attitude.

Make sure you have enough good food ready and waiting because I don't want you to be tempted to eat some takeout food and chips or chocolate. Planning to have healthy, nutritious food available is part of the planning process that helps you hit your target.

Remember NO EXCUSES, so treat it like a military operation and do your preparation.

WORKOUT JOURNAL

To make the most of your workout, keep track of the following:

WORK OUT: Note on which days and at what time you worked out. It is also great to keep track of how much effort it took to stay in the fight!

MOOD: Make note of how you're feeling before and after your workout.

TARGET: Have a set goal for each workout.

FOOD DIARY: Keep a daily food journal of all food and beverages consumed.

WEIGH IN: This should be done at the same time and day each week and in the same clothing.

Remember: It is okay to have a night out once in a while, but don't get carried away, this is a **NO EXCUSES** plan!

MONDAY	TUESDAY	WEDNESDAY	THURSDAY	FRIDAY	SATURDAY	SUNDAY
Weigh-in: 155 lbs. *6 am—aerobics* *Hard to get out of bed—very tired* *Worked out 45 minutes* *Breakfast: coffee; cereal w/ banana* *Lunch: turkey sand. on wheat, lt. mayo, lettuce, tomato; apple; cranberry juice* *Snack: granola bar* *Dinner: grilled salmon; salad*	*Breakfast: coffee; english muffin w/ jelly* *Lunch: vegetable soup; cranberry juice* *Snack: apple* *Dinner: whole wheat linguine with sautéed vegetables*	*Breakfast: coffee; fruit & yogurt* *Lunch: 1 slice pizza; soda* *Snack: no snack today!* *Dinner: chicken caesar salad* *7 pm—spin class Didn't want to go but felt bad about eating pizza. Felt great afterward— glad I went!*	*6 am—aerobics Easier to get out of bed today* *Worked out 45 minutes* *Breakfast: coffee; cereal w/ banana* *Lunch: turkey sand. on wheat, lt. mayo, lettuce, tomato; orange; skim milk* *Snack: a few almonds* *Dinner: grilled chicken w/ BBQ sauce; corn on cob (no butter)*	*Breakfast: coffee; fruit & yogurt* *Lunch: chicken salad wrap* *Dinner: ate out; Chinese food; steamed chicken rice and mixed vegetables with garlic sauce on the side. Did pretty well!*	*7 am—met Jane for brisk walk in park, 1 hour; felt great to have company!* *Breakfast: scrambled Egg Beaters, turkey bacon, OJ* *Lunch: tossed salad w/ grilled chicken* *Snack: grapes, yogurt* *Dinner: grilled lean steak, broccoli & cauliflower, baked sweet potato*	*Breakfast: strawberry smoothie* *Lunch: turkey burger, pasta salad* *Snack: carrot sticks* *Dinner: roasted pork tenderloin, couscous, green bean medley*

At the end of the week, assess how the week went, repeat after me: **OOH RAH!** and get ready to schedule your next week! Keep it going and make some money.

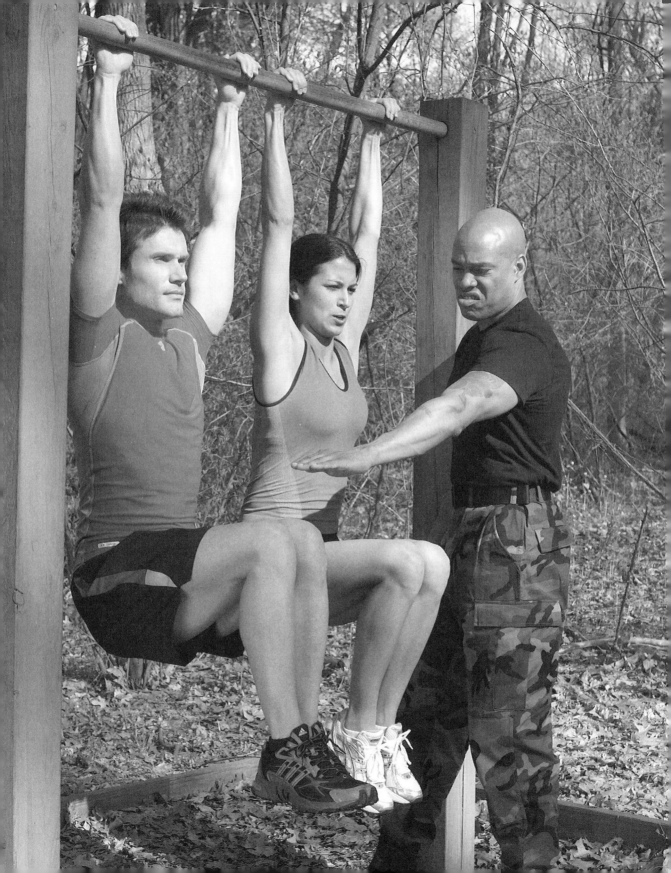

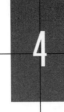

4

FINDING THE TIME— SUCKING IT UP!

Ever since I started appearing on television in the United States and Europe, motivating celebs on *Celebrity Fit Club,* I get stopped on the street and receive hundreds of e-mails about how people want to get fit and create a better body shape, something they can be proud of.

But I guess some ninety-five percent say: "It's great, Harvey, I want to do it, but I'm just so busy I don't have time. I can't fit it into my busy schedule."

You know what I'm going to say to that—it starts with a B . . . and ends with a T.

It's just a great big fat EXCUSE. And we don't have no excuses here. Right?

Of course we've all got hectic lifestyles. We've all got to go to work, look after the kids, see our parents and friends, go to the movies, and eat out.

Oh, and watch TV. That's what a lot of people do. They just flop down in front of the box and pick away at some food from the cupboard without even thinking about what they are eating.

Or they sit themselves in front of the computer and surf the Net, thinking they are doing something good.

Look, I know you've gotta watch some TV shows, I'm freakin' on one, ain't I? Of course my show is a good one because it's inspirational, and you can learn a heck of a lot of fitness tips and get motivated by watching all those overweight, unhealthy stars getting their stuff together, or on occasion, not, and that's because they make EXCUSES, too.

workout. How many people sit around watching *Grey's Anatomy* for at least a half an hour?

That's all it takes. Do the 30 and then you can sit down and chill and feel good about yourself. And as I've said, once you've gotten into these moves, then you can watch TV at the same time.

But you mustn't let yourself get too engrossed in that show, because otherwise you won't be working hard enough and that's important too, as you will

Are your life and health not worth 30 or 60 minutes of exercise?

And I hate EXCUSES.

EXCUSES just don't exist in my vocabulary. It's a dirty word.

So let's wipe that horrible, negative, loser word right out of our heads and say instead: "Heck, I'm really busy with my life, but I'm gonna make thirty minutes to spend time with Harvey and get myself together."

I can guarantee if I take a good, long look at your life I'd find you more than enough time to fit in this 30-minute

see from the plan over weeks and months as the intensity increases to continue to burn off that flab.

What about the excuse that you have to go to work to pay the bills? Time spent at work is the other biggest thing I hear. And it's trash.

Look, if you don't get that body moving and do some physical work and start eating better, you are going to be six feet under and put the responsibility of paying your bills on someone else, which is a pretty crappy way of living (and dying).

Take control. It's your life, your body, your family. It's all in *your* hands.

I know, it's sooo easy to be lazy and take the path of the least resistance, but what I'm saying is fight to get yourself out of that comfort zone and move up a few gears. We've all got it in us.

People say they haven't got time to go to the gym or they can't afford the fees.

Well, that's no excuse (that word again, yugghh) because my answer to you is that I have specifically designed this plan so that you don't have to leave your house if you don't want to.

It's all here, nice and easy and in manageable chunks, and it won't cost you a cent, only a few minutes of your time.

And I can also guarantee that, on average, you are going to grab back that time by living not only longer but with better quality of life.

We can't cheat diseases and illnesses and accidents, but we can put the odds slightly more in our favor by making our minds and bodies stronger.

Everything here (I have included some machine work for those with access to fitness equipment) can be done 3 inches from your sofa and can be done by men and women of all ages (get that checkup first, of course).

If it all goes well, you'll get the health bug, and I sincerely hope you do. Otherwise, I might have to pay you a house call. Once you get the health bug, you'll be more motivated to go down to your local gym to work out on the machines.

What I foresee is that you will get into the groove with these exercises and become addicted to feeling good about yourself and feeling good about the way other folk look at you.

Don't think that you're gonna become a monk or something. You aren't gonna become a recluse or an exercise freak with bulging biceps and thunderous thighs.

You'll just be a better balanced human being who wants to enjoy life, because that's what life is for. Let's face it, no one can maintain a perfect doggone diet all the time.

Like I said, I like the odd cigar and cognac. It's a treat. Once you get it under control and you are living a fit lifestyle, you'll be able to cheat and get right back on track. If you do things in moderation, that is exercise, diet, and

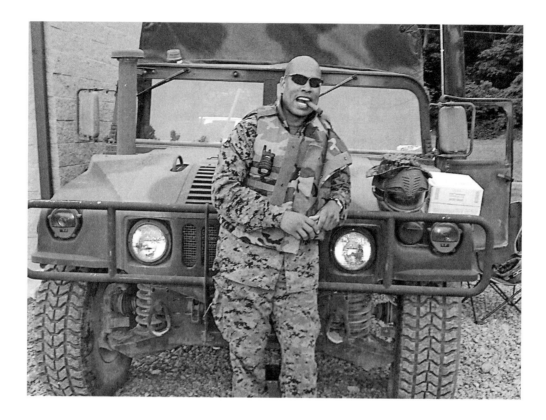

the occasional beer or two, we're gonna get you there.

My little secret vice is cheesecake. I love the damn stuff and when I see it on a menu, I find it hard to resist.

It's one of the few sweet things I go for. Otherwise I really don't touch desserts.

I was out with friends in New York recently and I saw a lady nearby having the cheesecake. I just had to have a slice of it.

But when it came I had just two forkfuls and left the rest. That was enough for me. My friends said, "Harvey, what's wrong, isn't it good?"

I said it was delicious, but I had had my fill. It was sufficient. I'd had the taste and didn't need any more. It may have been a waste of good food, and that's a shame, but I'm also a portion-control man, so I like to keep it in shape on my plate too.

That's a major bugbear for me. Overeating. I'm not a trained dietician, but I will later share my views on diet, and my approach has served my family and me well. But basically I think it's like life. Keep it as simple as possible because other elements are sure as hell gonna make it complicated somewhere along the way.

So, as you know, I like small portions, not huge platefuls of stuff. And those portions should be as fat-free, salt-free, and sugar-free as possible.

Go fresh as often as you can. Knock out the candy and chips and fries when

dly and can become a bit obsessive. I just say eat sensibly and try to eat healthily. Watch how much you put on your plate. You will be surprised how far a lot less will go.

There's nothing wrong with eating five times a day if you want. Just make sure it's good stuff.

The thing I really love to snack on is a nice, juicy green apple. Nothing better. Try it. It works.

I'll give you some other ideas down the line.

I also think that if you are moving

Win the battle today and set yourself up for winning the war against fat and obesity.

you can. Go for fruit instead. Watch the dairy products, but go for some quality yogurts. Drink lots of water. Chuck the soda down the drain. Natural cereals and nuts are good. Beware of too much processed food. Take a look at labels and get used to rejecting items that are too high in the elements I have mentioned.

This isn't a calorie-counting program. I think that's too fussy and fid-

much more energetically than you were, you will start to burn off the calories and shed the pounds.

It is important to realize that by eating well, rather than being full of sugary crap, you will have more energy and it will be released gradually as you need it. In effect, your body will be working as it should be. What we are trying to achieve here is balance.

Right now you are out of balance and probably feeling a little heavy and sluggish for all the reasons I mentioned above.

Obesity is all around us, and the United States is famous for it. We are the unhealthiest country on earth. And parts of Europe, especially Britain, aren't far behind.

Let's go to war on obesity, and in doing so, let's get ourselves in shape.

I suggest that people should do my fitness plan four times a week, but once in a while, it is probably okay to miss one of the workouts and replace it with an energetic night—or day, if you fancy it. This is supposed to be a fun sex session with your partner, of course.

I guarantee that your interest in this activity will increase quite sharply after a few weeks into the fight. You will be feeling better about yourself, you won't be quite so big in those normally unseen places, and you WILL have more energy, that's a promise.

So not only are you getting a new lease on life here, you're also getting a brand-new sex life, and that's gonna do wonders for your relationship. Your lust levels are going to rocket.

It'll be like meeting your loved one for the first time all over again. Remember the excitement of those first bouts of passion with your new girlfriend or boyfriend?

Well, you've just gone and lit the fuse again, and there's no way of telling how good that's gonna be.

It's all part of being in better shape and sending healthy hormones racing around your veins. Man, you're gonna be glowing with vigor and vitality.

So this is a reward system as well. By getting rid of that gut and those bat wings, you're gonna increase your love life without the aids of those little chemical pills.

All that fresh, raw power coursing through your body. Makes you want to turn to the exercise pages right now, doesn't it?

If that's not motivational, I don't know what is.

I must admit I got a little freaked when a guy got in touch with me to say his wife had pinned a picture of me to the headboard of their marital bed.

He said it was because his wife had been having difficulty getting out of bed in the morning to do her exercises, so she stuck the photo there to motivate her to get up and get to it.

I thought the guy was going to shoot me or kick my ass or something really bad because there she was, looking at me to get her going.

But the dude said he wanted to shake my hand and thank me because since the picture got put there he was having the best sex of his life; he'd never known it better and it was all due to his wife working out, having more energy than ever, and getting in the mood for love.

Whatever turns you on, I guess!

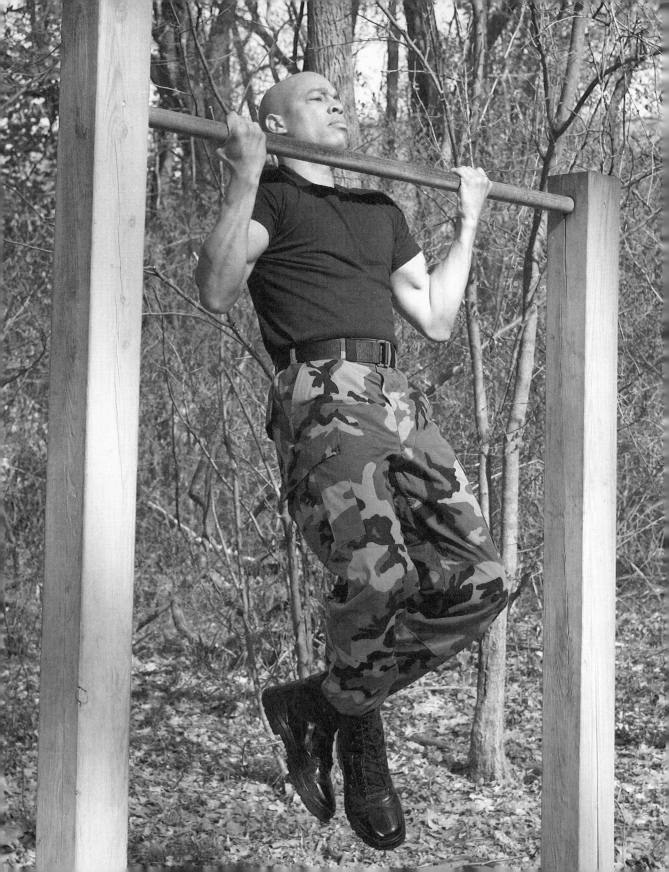

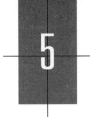

MARINE READY

I put together Harvey Walden's No Excuses! Fitness Workout as a result of being a drill instructor in the U.S. Marines—the toughest fighting force in the world.

Marines have the hardest boot camp in existence. It's the most challenging and the longest. That's why we call ourselves "the few, the proud, the Marines." Because not everyone can make it.

For me this fight against obesity started in the Marine Corps. That was where I first dreamed up the No Excuses! honing and toning, one-stop workout you're reading now—to make my marines the fittest, strongest, smartest recruits in the whole doggone company.

So if you do this workout and shape up the Harvey Walden way, you'll be following in the footsteps of all those marines. And that's an accomplishment anyone can be proud of.

Staying motivated means always wanting to be the best you can be. Better than anyone else—the best of all. Your best self.

I always knew I wanted to be the best. And I was stubborn.

I was proud to graduate from drill-instructor school. The day I walked across that stage I said to myself: "Holy shit, you have done this outstanding thing, and now you will have an impact on and influence other people's lives and make marines." When they put that "Smokey Bear" on my head I knew this was it, and it was time to go to work.

So when I got my first platoon at age 28, I was the new kid on the block and right away I started looking for how to work my way to the top. I'd always been an overachiever and a perfectionist, and I wanted to prove myself.

New drill instructors have to do all the errands for the platoon. They keep you running morning till night learning all the ropes. You do the paperwork, find out how the laundry gets done, how the platoon operates, what makes it tick. You are the lowest on the pole.

That was NOT where I wanted to be.

There are four drill instructors for each platoon of 88 recruits, with a senior drill instructor in control. I was at the bottom—the fourth-hat Nick. New drill instructors are called Nicks after the 24-hour TV channel, Nickelodeon. As the new drill instructor, you work your butt off 18 hours every day. It isn't 24, but it sure as hell feels like it.

In the marines, we call it "working the trenches."

I didn't give a rat's ass. I knew I could work hard. But I wanted to win. And win fast. Without wasting time.

So while I was running errands, I took the chance to sneak around the other platoons to see what they were doing. I watched their PT (physical training) and how they were training, so that I could figure out how to beat them.

I saw I could beat them through training, so that's what I decided to do: make my platoon the strongest and fittest of all.

At the end of the day at boot camp, you get what we call "square away time." The senior drill instructors go home, and they leave you, the fourth hat, with the boys overnight. That was my time; I was in charge, and even my senior drill instructor didn't know that I was taking half an hour of downtime every night to do circuit training right there in the squad bay (living quarters) where we slept.

That was the very beginning of Harvey Walden's No Excuses! Fitness Workout, right there in that squad bay, out on the island.

I made sure none of the other platoons knew what we were up to. It was a secret. I always sent a couple of recruits to have a shower first, and then posted them as sentries. I didn't want anyone to know about my spec-ops (special operations). To really kick ass we needed the surprise factor too.

So the whole workout was done in silence. I used hand and arm signals to give instructions, rotating my fingers to tell them to begin. It kept the guys motivated and it kept their eyes on me.

decline push-ups in between the foot lockers, and leg lifts, and stepping on the lockers, up and down.

At the end I'd say to them: "Think about the money we made today. It's serving a purpose. Tomorrow, watch how much better you'll be."

You better believe I was right. After just two weeks there was a difference. We started getting the highest Physi-

Hey, I need 110% from you. If you have a bad hair day 10% of you is already gone so I'm making up for it now.

I used what I had in the squad bay for the workout, and I didn't have a whole lot. All each man had was that goddamn foot locker and his own couple of square feet of space to get fit. So there I was, devising a routine for working out right there in that few feet of space.

I started with a series of calisthenics—dips—and incline push-ups, leaning on the foot locker, flutter kicks,

cal Fitness Test (PFT) scores in the company. We kept working out. We kept those scores. And they got better. "You're warriors," I told them. "You're going to win the pugilistics," and they did. They started winning everything, because they were strong—still doing PT in the morning, doing secret spec-ops with me at night, making money.

That was how I moved straight up to the top. It was unheard of, but I did it.

My commanding officer called me into his office. I thought I was in trouble, but he said to me: "We're making

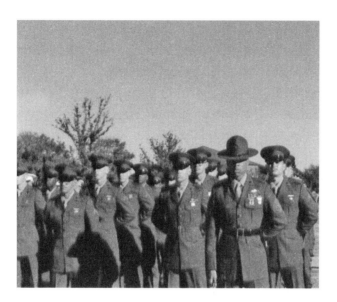

tlebutt, that they'd set me up to pull me down, but I proved them wrong. When they saw what I was doing they soon got over their jealousy.

Once I had my own platoon to train I was motivated to win, so everything I did with those recruits had to serve a purpose. It wasn't just the spec-ops workout. I would make sure we got the drill basics down

you a senior drill instructor. You're professional, smart, and I think you're ready. Can you handle it?"

"Yes, I can handle it, sir," I said.

It was a big challenge and big pressure to move from the bottom of the pile straight to senior drill instructor. There were guys who had been waiting two years for that chance and I had only been there a few months; yet here I was, in the fight, competing with others and running my own doggone platoon.

The thing at the back of my mind was that I wouldn't get support from the other hats. There was a lot of jealousy at first. I heard some of the scut-

picture perfect. I was always intense and gave attention to detail.

I never bullshitted. Those kids, they were Generation X, and I knew they were smart. Other drill instructors had other styles, but for me, my message to them was always: "Be responsible. The way you walk, the way you stand, something you do on the PT field, it all serves a *purpose*. Everything you learn here will make you a better marine. Hey, I'm teaching you how to be the best warrior and stay alive out there if you're in combat."

I was shooting for the moon, which meant even if I failed, I would still hit the stars.

These young marines would leave the island never forgetting how they were shaped into the marines and the people that they became. Some went on to become officers, politicians, and successful businessmen, and to this day they still have the great memories of how their drill instructor helped them achieve that in some way. Now that I'm on TV, I often get e-mails from prior recruits. They come from all walks of life and they're doing great things, but they still tell the war stories of boot camp and tell me how I taught them how to be a marine and a man.

When people see me on TV, they often assume I'm an actor, not a marine. They don't realize that I'm the real deal, that I've been right there in the fight.

A few weeks ago a guy got in touch to say he was in the bathroom when he heard my voice on TV. He stopped brushing his teeth and he came into the room.

"That's Drill Instructor Walden," he said to his wife.

"No it's not. It's Harvey," she said. But he was not mistaken. He remembered me from his weeks at boot camp, and when he contacted me he told me that my voice still haunts him today. That man is at NASA now.

So this is why I KNOW there are NO excuses. This fitness routine worked for the marines, and it will work for you. It will make you fit and healthy and toned and attractive, and it will give you purpose and pride and a sense of accomplishment. And you will be able to walk tall and live your life knowing you are the best you can be.

I always knew I wanted to be the best. We can all prove ourselves. That's what it's about. Life's a challenge, and the choice is yours. Are you going to sit back on your butt and ruin your life, or get up and turn it around?

All the way through my time as a drill instructor I did the spec-ops workout with my platoons. It made us money, it gave us the edge that made my platoons win, it got us where we wanted to be. That can happen for you, too, if you follow these routines and make NO EXCUSES.

Think how you'll feel when you've got that toned body. Think how you'll feel when you're healthy and alert all the time. Get to your goal and reward yourself. Or mirror your workout with a buddy and agree to reward each other. Find your inner motivator and put it to work on becoming the best.

Stay active. Go the extra mile. You're going to win because you're making that secret effort that puts you ahead of the others. I know—it worked for my marines.

Find things to do that get you moving. You know what they are. Do what you like best. Running or walking, yard work or housework, dancing or romancing, if you move your body, believe me, you're making money.

You can do the workout in the yard or the park if you prefer. I first started taking marines outside when I got to London and had a company of three platoons. We were a security force taking care of the U.S. Embassy in Grosvenor Square. One platoon always had to guard the building, one was at Eastcote, and one was held back as a reactionary force.

To protect that building those guys had to be strong, and to get strong, they had to get out of their comfort zone.

You often see people in the gym on the treadmill, just taking it easy, nice and slow. I'm saying: Get out of your comfort zone. You need to try something you wouldn't dream of attempting, an accomplishment that makes you feel you can take on anything.

My signature moves will take you to that place. And those moves will make you think: *Hey, I did something that real marines do.*

With the workouts in the park, I was trying to build endurance and stamina. Those guys needed it: It was essential. They had to be able to run up and down stairs, with a vest and pistol belt on—and a bullet-proof vest is heavy. They had to be able to *move*. I had to make sure they were in shape.

So out at Eastcote we would start from base and do an Indian run all the way to the park. This was running in a long column, me at the front, until I'd say: "Kick it!" and the guy at the back had to sprint all the way to the front and take over, and so on, until we worked all the way through the line.

After starting with a good run, I'd lay out laminated cards with the exercises in a big circle, and everyone had to take up a station and exercise in that place until I'd whistle. Then they'd run around the whole circle and end up at a different station.

To vary it, we'd do "suicide sit-ups," where you do as many crunches as you can in 2 minutes, then in 1 minute 30 seconds, then in 1 minute, and then in 30 seconds—and then the same with push-ups. And I was shooting for 100 crunches in the 2 minutes. Sometimes I made it harder for them, like making them clap between push-ups. They did it well, and it brought up their PFT scores until the CO was really impressed.

a lot of energy. It was hard on my legs, especially because I had football practice on Thursdays and Sundays too.

I put everything in there, to dig deep and do something different from the average trainer.

That was why I also invented a couple of signature moves, the exclamation marks of the workout—the wow! that makes you feel good.

The Grasshopper Harvey Builders with Arm Rotations in Stage Two have that wow! factor. This exercise will make you feel good about how far you've come once you get to it. Your

You need to try something you wouldn't dream of attempting, an accomplishment that makes you feel you can take on anything.

I would time it so that each platoon worked out three times a week. But it wore me out, because I was doing it every day.

So I'd get up at 5 a.m. and go to the gym to try to get some lifting in and bulk up some muscle, because all that running and working out was burning

average fit person has a hard time with this one. The way I do it means more arm rotations, so you're really getting the burn, but it builds upper body strength and strength in your arms. It's a good total body workout, and it helps your abdominal muscles as well.

The Hard-Core Harvey Builders with Arm Rotations in Stage Three was a move I invented one rainy day in a hotel room in Myrtle Beach. It's hard core because it's based on a tough move I used to do with the marines. The Hard-Core Harvey Builders in this workout are easier, but they will make you feel like you're really making money—as well as having a good time.

In all these moves, you're using your

So it wasn't about winning this time. And I didn't have to do secret in-house circuit training anymore.

OCS was about peak condition—in body as well as mind.

We had to stay fighting fit and ready for anything, so suicide sit-ups and pull-ups in the squad bay stayed on the menu. These were guys who were having to write essays on leadership when they messed up, instead of doing push-

Move out of that comfort zone and don't stop when you hit the wall.

own body weight all the time, so it's the perfect amount of resistance for you to get well-toned without bulking up too much.

When I got back to the United States after London, I went right into Office Candidate School (OCS) as a drill instructor. Instead of training warriors, we were training people to be responsible; we were preparing them for leadership. They had to be very, very smart, able to make good decisions, and inspire respect.

ups. They needed brain skills as well as muscle, but the muscle was important too. If you're not physically fit, how can you be mentally fit?

For the first two weeks the commander was evaluating those officers, assessing their leadership and time-management skills.

But to keep them steady I made sure their PT in the morning was very intense. I ran those guys till they dog-gone puked. We got right down and did push-ups and recon pulls. When they graduated, they were going into officer positions so they had to be as near perfect as a man can be. And they got there. They did it.

That's why I KNOW this workout is worth the effort.

Thousands of marines have proved it over more than 200 years. They were motivated by the desire to serve their country and flag and to be the best they could be. They were inspired by the desire to survive and to be proud of what they'd accomplished. They wanted to stand tall with honor and say: They are the few, the proud.

You can be proud too. Find a motivator that works for you. Move out of that comfort zone and don't stop when you hit the wall. Go right through and shoot for the moon, just like the marines.

And if you miss, you'll still hit the stars.

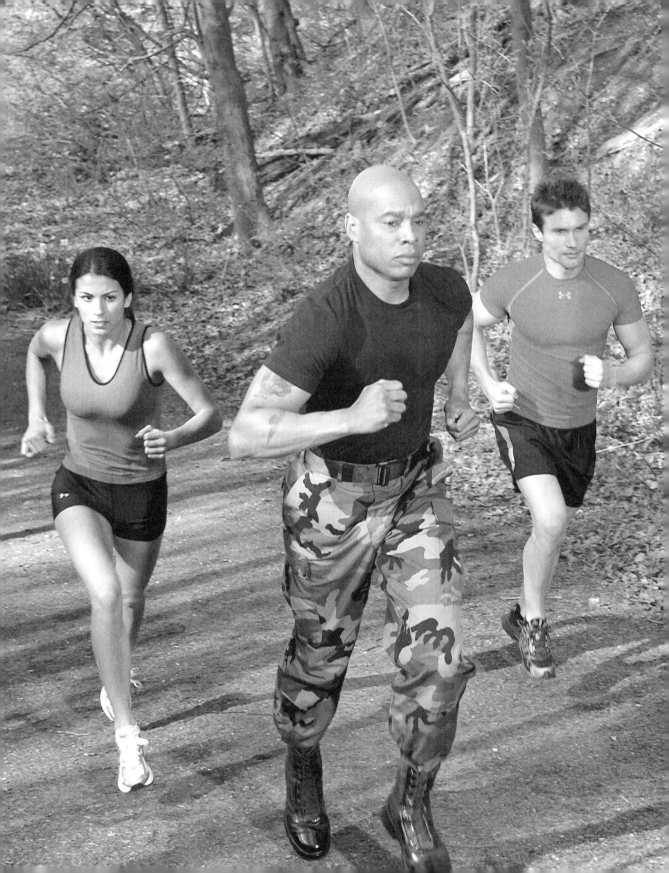

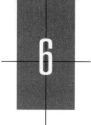

THE HARVEY WALDEN STAGES TO TOTAL BODY FITNESS

So here we are, ready to kick ass and get into the fight. You will see a difference within just a few weeks if you follow this program.

Even doing the first plan will give you a more toned body. You'll burn calories and feel fit, your self-esteem will be lifted, and you'll start feeling better and looking better. And look out if you're doggone male; the women are going to be all over you. Is your life not worth 30 minutes of your time four times a week?

So you plan your day and you keep your diary, as we've said before, being honest with yourself, and you get to the point where you make a commitment. And you say: "I'm gonna wake up tomorrow and I'm gonna work out."

The motivation comes from within yourself if you've found your motivating factor, but you can also get together with other people and do this in a group. That way, you motivate one another to follow this half-hour road to total body fitness.

And remember: This is something you CAN do. You get into the fight and you start. When you've done your workout you look back and you think, *Wow, I've accomplished something,* and that's where your self-esteem is boosted. And your confidence is boosted in the fight against obesity.

It only seems tough because we're trying to come out of the comfort zone. That's always an effort.

We all have to pull ourselves out of the comfort zone to achieve. Every now and then I have to pull myself out of it too. I know how it feels. We can

USE A STOPWATCH

The workouts are all based on the 30-second or 1-minute timings at Levels 1, 2 and 3, so you do need to get yourself a timing device.

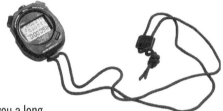

Don't avoid this, grasshoppers. It's part of the deal, so get your ass over to the mall and you'll know you're doing it right. A timer keeps you honest and it means you can give me 110% of your commitment.

You can buy a proper stopwatch in any sports store and it will last you a long time. Or if you can't find a stopwatch, just get hold of a cheap regular wristwatch, like a Timex, that includes a countdown feature. You set the timer to 30 seconds or 1 minute, and it beeps when you're done.

When I used to do suicide situps with the marines, I'd set the countdown all the way up to two minutes, and they had to carry right on until they heard that beep.

Even if you're watching your favorite TV show while you're working out, that beep will cut through the sound and you'll know your time's up.

When I do fitness clinics, I'm the one who holds the watch. But when I used to do these workouts myself in the barrack room, I just set my wristwatch. All I had to do was set the timer, do the exercise, and when I heard it beep, I just hit Reset and went again for the next 30 seconds.

So it's simple. And that means there's NO excuse.

be happy and content and keep plodding along, but when we have to change, it's tough. So sometimes you just have to shock your life with something different.

WHY YOU NEED TO WARM UP

You've got to warm up. No excuses. I've put a warm-up program right at the beginning of each plan, because you have to do that every time. There is a cooldown too. It's an essential part of exercising in a safe and healthy way.

In this program, you keep moving all the time, so you begin by marching on the spot.

Why? Because marching on the spot puts you into a good low-down first gear. It starts your pulse and heart off working gently, and it gives your body time to adjust to what you're going to do. It sets you up for the next exercise. It also maximizes your calorie burn because you keep moving all the time.

What a lot of people need to do is just move. Just walking to the doggone grocery store, for someone who's overweight, is going to start dropping the pounds. Just moving!

A lot of times even in the gym you'll see people sitting around and wasting time between exercises, or standing there watching the TV. In my workout, you don't do that. It's designed to keep you moving so you can keep burning the fat. While you're looking at the page and thinking, *Okay, what am I doing next?* and, *I've got X minutes left,* your heart rate is staying up.

So in this workout, whether marching or, in the later stages, jogging on the spot, you ALWAYS keep moving.

Throughout the workout, the marching goes from first, to second, to third gear.

So start marching gently, well within your range. Move to the steam engines exercise and try to get the coordination right. It will help your balance, and it's part of me being a little bit humorous. You see some people doing this exercise and it makes you laugh, keeps the workout interesting and helps your mind relax.

Gears are part of the transition between exercises, like driving a car. Just like you shift in a car to second gear, you're going to be moving a little bit faster and doing more repetitions or steps when you move up a gear in your marching.

It's up to you how quickly you take it, as long as you go just a little bit quicker when you change up. And don't stop moving.

If you get a little out of breath, that's okay. Being breathless means you're working out. The only time you should stop is if you're feeling light-headed.

WE ARE IN THE FIGHT AGAINST OBESITY AND WE ARE NOT GOING TO STOP UNTIL WE KICK ASS.

STAGE ONE:

GET OFF YOUR BUTT

MARCH ON THE SPOT
(1 MINUTE)

Feet are shoulder-width apart, hands at sides, and you begin to pick up your feet ankle high and pump arms simultaneously.

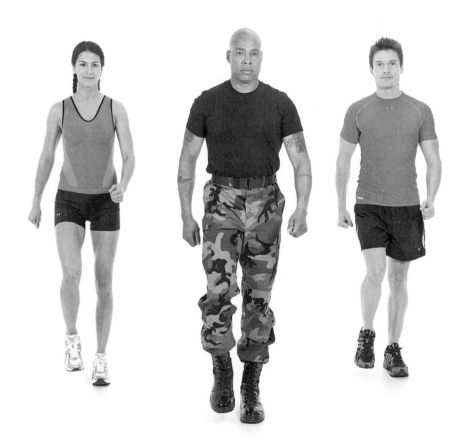

STEAM ENGINES
(1 MINUTE)

Stand with feet shoulder-width apart and place your hands behind your ears. Start by lifting the left foot up, bringing the knee in front of you, and at the same time keeping your hands behind your ears while bringing the right elbow down and across to touch the right elbow to the left knee. Then repeat on the opposite side.

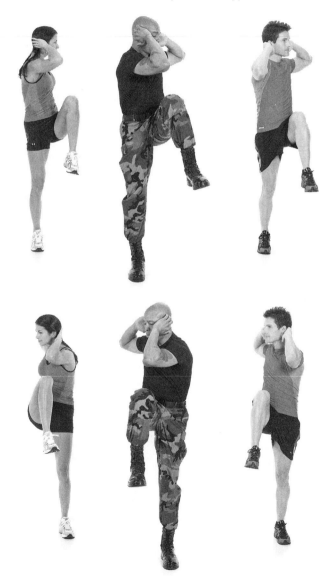

SIDE STRADDLE HOP

Start with your feet together and your hands at your side. Jump outward and land with both feet wider than shoulder-width apart while swinging your arms outward and up until your hands meet over your head. Reverse these actions as you jump back to the starting position.

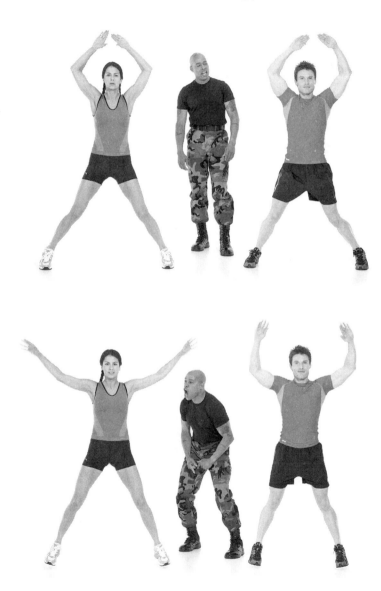

NECK STRETCH

Standing with feet shoulder-width apart, lean your head to the left, stretching the right side. Hold for a count of 10, switch, and repeat.

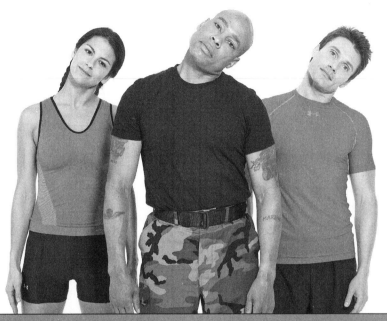

Welcome to Stretching

You have to do stretches before the workout so that you loosen and get the blood flowing into your muscles, gently getting your pulse up. You'll be tempted to gaff off. Don't. Stretching helps your muscles get a bit more flexible, and that helps you get the most out of the workout.

For example, if I'm working my triceps and I can't even get my arm out in front of me, stretching will give me more flexibility. It won't help build muscles, but it's essential for health and tone, and it helps with flexibility and recovery.

I've given you a lot of stretches to cover and they'll get you going! There's no stopping now.

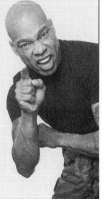

After a workout you always have to stretch as well. Never ever miss it. When you stretch your muscles, it helps them recover. If you don't do it, you'll be tight the next day, and you're gonna be sore. If you don't want to be sore, you'd better do stretches!

TRICEPS STRETCH

Stand with your feet shoulder-width apart. Bend the left elbow and place your left hand between your shoulder blades. Gently pull the left elbow with the right hand. Hold for a count of 10. Switch arms and repeat.

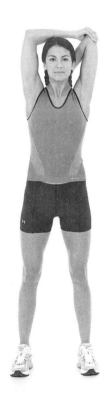
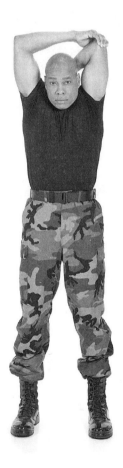
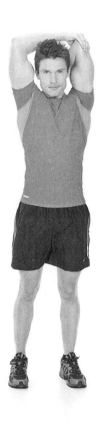

SHOULDER STRETCH

Stand with your feet shoulder-width apart. Bring your left arm across your chest and give a gentle pull with the right hand. Hold for a count of 10. Switch arms and repeat.

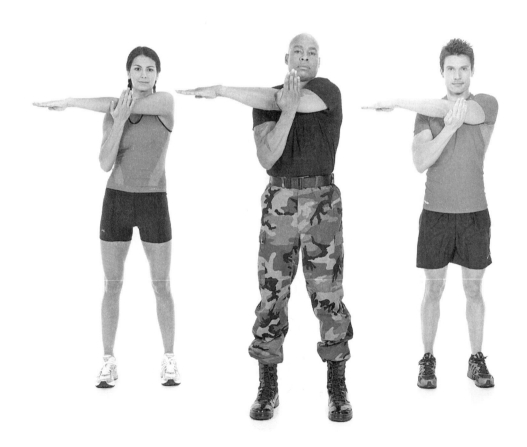

>>>>> **CHEST STRETCH** Stand with your feet shoulder-width apart. Clasp hands together behind the lower back with palms facing up. Pull arms toward the sky and hold for a count of 10. >>>>>

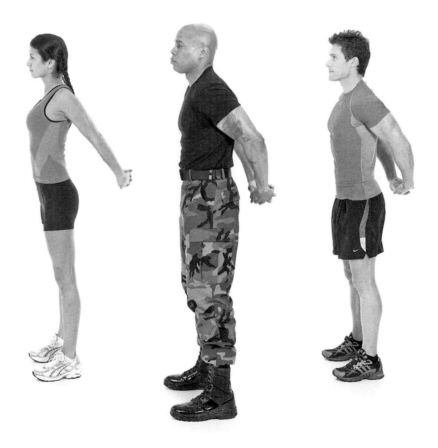

UPPER BACK STRETCH

Stand with your feet shoulder-width apart. Extend your arms in front of you at shoulder height with hands clasped and palms facing away from you. Push arms forward, rounding upper back while bending your knees slightly. Hold for a count of 10.

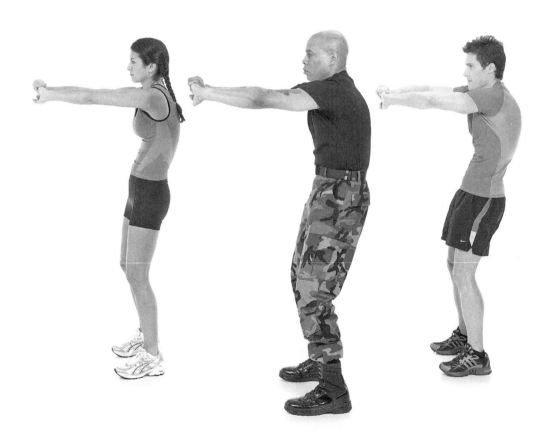

HAMSTRING STRETCH

Lie on your back. Bring your left knee straight toward your chest, grasping the left leg below the knee. The right knee should be slightly bent and the right foot remains on the floor. Hold for a count of 10. Switch legs and repeat.

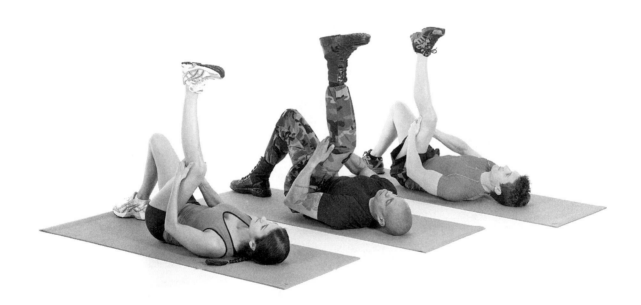

CALF STRETCH

Stand with your feet shoulder-width apart. Place your right foot in front of you, keeping both feet pointing forward and both heels on the floor. Bend the right knee slightly as you feel the stretch in the left calf. Hold for a count of 10. Switch legs and repeat.

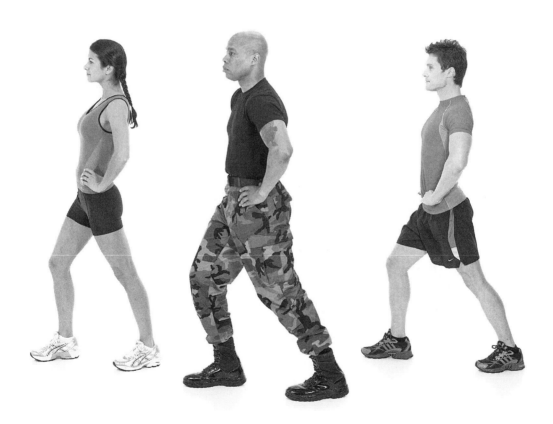

GROIN STRETCH

Sitting with both knees bent and bottoms of the feet together, grasp the feet and push your knees, with your elbows toward the floor. Hold for a count of 10.

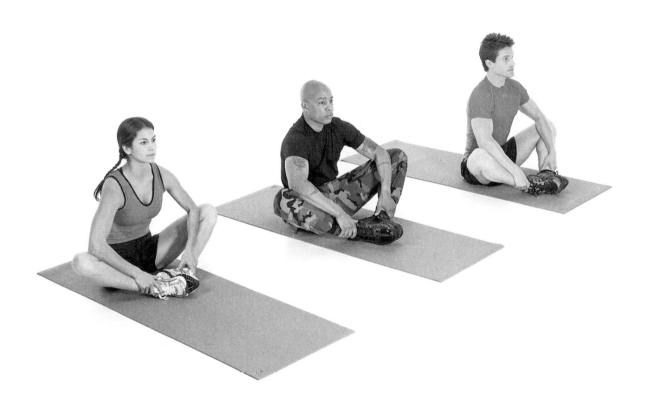

QUAD STRETCH

Lie on the floor on your right side. Grab the left ankle with the left hand and pull the left knee straight back. Hold for a count of 10. Switch legs and repeat.

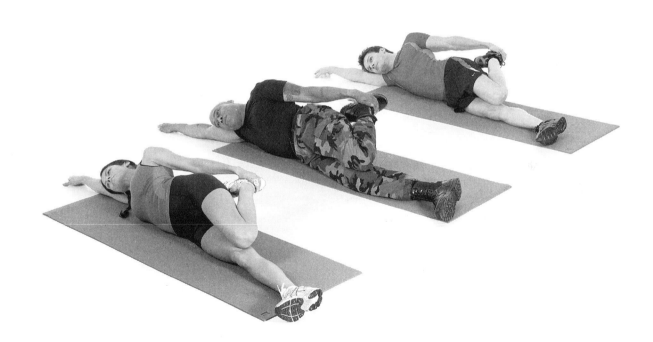

LOW BACK STRETCH

Lie on your back. Bring left knee toward your chest with your right leg remaining on the floor. Hold for a count of 10. Switch legs and repeat.

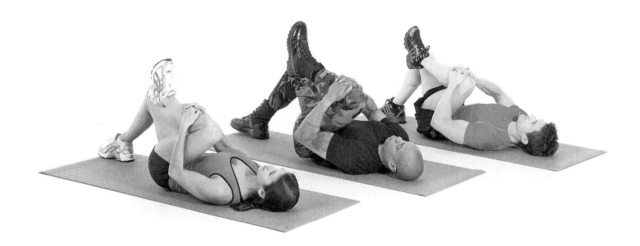

MARCH ON THE SPOT
(30 SECONDS)

Feet are shoulder-width apart, hands at sides, and you begin to pick up your feet ankle high and pump arms simultaneously.

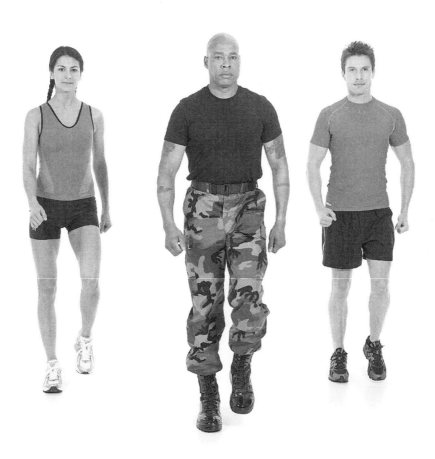

SIDE STRADDLE HOP

Start with your feet together and your hands at your sides. Jump outward and land with both feet wider than shoulder-width apart, while swinging your arms outward and up until your hands meet over your head. Reverse these actions as you jump back to the starting position.

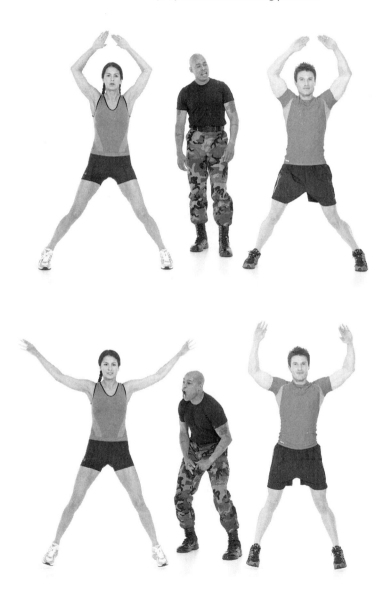

MARCH ON THE SPOT
(30 SECONDS)

Your feet are shoulder-width apart with your hands at your sides. Start with your left foot and march in place, alternating picking up each foot about ankle high. Pump your arms simultaneously.

SCISSOR JACK

Similar to cross-country skiing but without the ski poles and skis.

Scissor jack is about sliding, and you should take it slow and do it for the full 30 seconds. Even people who have never exercised before will find it fun, and everyone can do it.

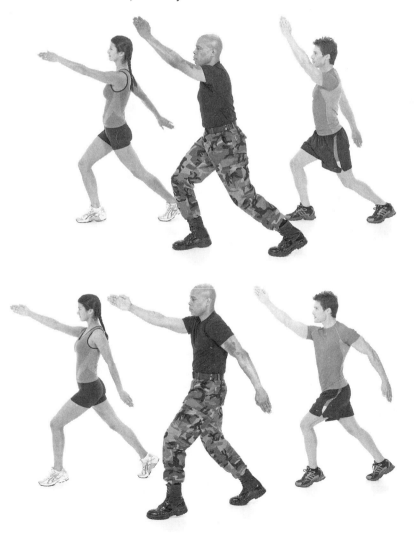

MARCH ON THE SPOT (1ST GEAR) »»»»»»»»»»»»»»»»»»»»

HALF JACK

This starts in the same position as the side straddle hop. Spread your feet apart, but instead of your hands going above your head, your hands and arms will come only halfway up, until they are about shoulder height, with palms facing the floor.

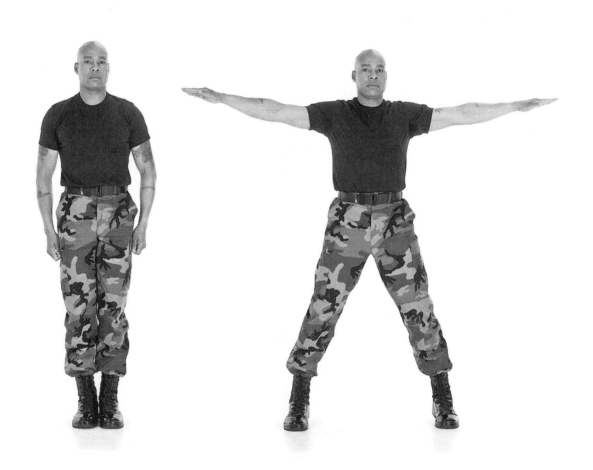

MARCH ON THE SPOT (1ST GEAR) »»»»»»»»»»»»»»»»»»

ARM ROTATIONS TO SIDE LATERAL FORWARD

Stand with your feet shoulder-width apart. Raise your arms until they are shoulder height, straight out to your sides with palms facing downward. Rotate in small circles forward.

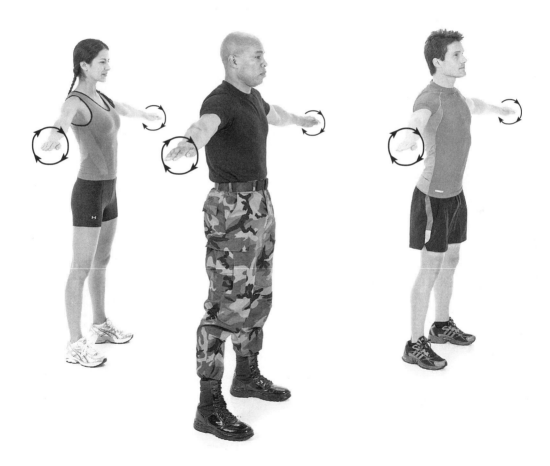

MARCH ON THE SPOT (2ND GEAR) >>

PUSH-UPS

Yes, you can start on your knees in Stage One!

Lie on your stomach with your hand placed under each shoulder and with your fingers extended and joined with your thumb along the hand. Push up while keeping your back straight and then lower yourself until your chest is about an inch or two off the floor, but do not let your body touch the floor. If you are doing your push-ups by using your knees, start by bending your knees and crossing your feet before you push off with your hands. Keep your feet in this crossed position, with your knees bent throughout the 30-second duration of the exercise.

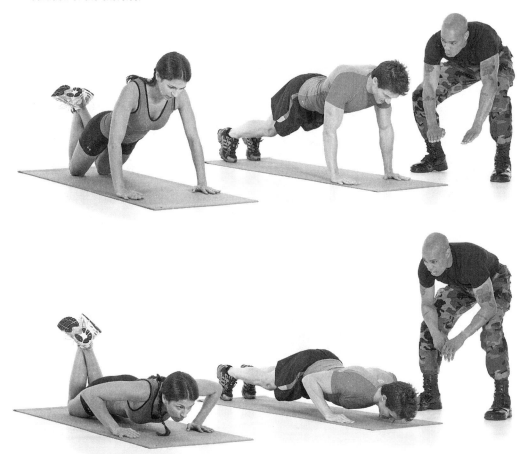

MOVE THE MAR

Welcome to Push-ups

I love push-ups. They're the ultimate core builder. They work everything right through the trunk of your body and help your balance. They're simple to do, and you need no equipment, just a floor and your own body weight. But if you do them right and do them enough, they will change your life and give you the best upper-body workout you can get outside a gym.

Push-ups make you stronger, build up your triceps, and work your chest muscles. Females will find their upper body is toned and shaped, their bosoms will be firmed up, and their backs and arms will slim and tone, which means good-bye to "bat wings." Push-ups can help get rid of the "man boobs" that so many people ask me about, too.

It's all in the push-ups, so do them right and do them often.

And watch your hand placement. If your hands are too far back or forward, that's bad for your rotator cuff. So look carefully at the pictures on this page and get it right. It's not just about how wide apart you place them; it's about positioning the depth.

Push-ups don't build musculature. They're not going to make women look like guys. For extra bulking, you need to be in a gym lifting heavy weights.

But push-ups do build core muscles, and if you diet too, and cut all the calories down, doing push-ups will make a big difference in how you look, because your body will be toned.

CHING UP ANOTHER GEAR.

MARCH ON THE SPOT (2ND GEAR) ›››››››››››››››››››››››››

DIAMOND PUSH-UPS
(YOU CAN USE YOUR KNEES DURING STAGE ONE.)

Lie on your stomach. Place your hands just under your chest with the index fingers of each hand and both thumbs touching, forming the shape of a diamond. All other fingers are extended. You will perform the exercise just as you would a normal push-up.

In the marines we do seven different kinds of push-ups before we go out on our runs. Can YOU do the Daily Seven?

1. Knee push-up
2. Regular push-up with normal grip
3. Diamond or tricep push-up
4. Wide grip push-up
5. Dive Bomber push-up
6. Push-up with clap
7. Incline push-up with feet up

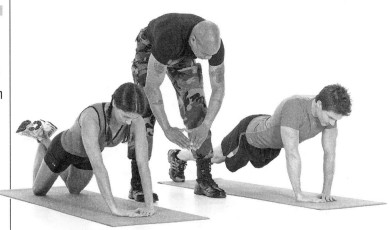

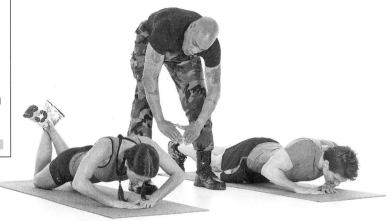

MARCH ON THE SPOT (2ND GEAR) >>> >>> >>> >>> >>> >>> >>> >>> >>>

WIDE PUSH-UPS
(YOU CAN USE YOUR KNEES DURING STAGE ONE.)

Lie on your stomach. Place your hands slightly wider than shoulder-width apart, with your fingers extended and each thumb joined along the hand. Push up while keeping your back straight, and then lower yourself until your chest is about an inch or two off the floor but do not let your body touch the floor. If you are doing your push-ups by using your knees, start by bending your knees and crossing your feet before you push off with your hands. Keep your feet in this crossed position, with your knees bent throughout the 30-second duration of the exercise.

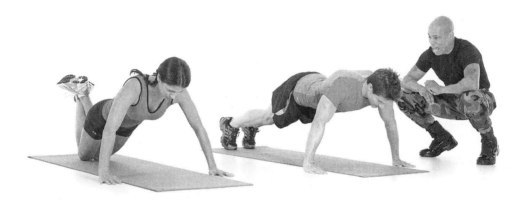

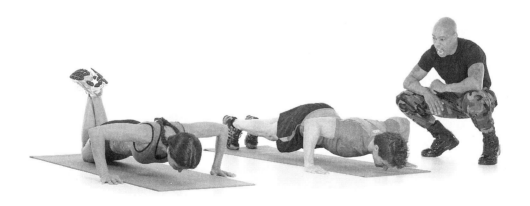

MARCH ON THE SPOT (2ND GEAR) »»»»»»»»»»»»»»»»»»

4-COUNT BEAT BOOT SQUATS: 3 DOWN, 1 UP

Stand with your feet shoulder-width apart. Extend your arms in front of the body at shoulder height. Squat down for three counts by bending the knees a little more at each level and keeping your belly button pulled in and your weight on your heels. On the third count, lower your hands to your sides and reach around and tap your ankles. Once ankles are tapped, you will stand completely up in one count while raising your arms so that they are again extended in front of you at shoulder height, completing one repetition of the exercise.

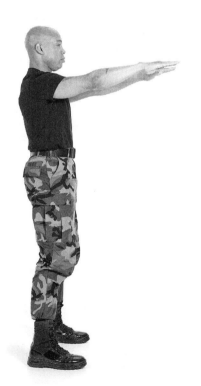
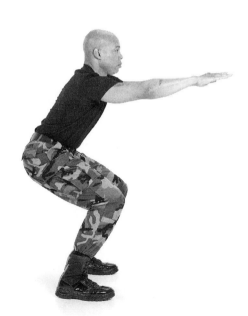

Beat boot squats are something I invented a long time ago, when my recruits were pissing me off in the marines. I used to say: "You're pissing me off, beat your damn boots!" and off they'd go, three counts up, three counts down. It was a way of teaching them discipline, but they were also getting a good workout and getting stronger. This exercise stabilizes and tones your calf muscles—as my recruits found out.

People often focus on thighs, which is where fat tends to gather in women—with men it's the gut—but it's important to work your calf muscles too.

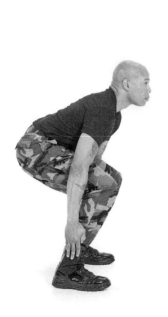
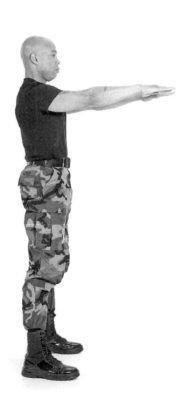

MARCH ON THE SPOT (2ND GEAR) ≫≫≫≫≫≫≫≫≫≫≫≫≫≫≫≫≫≫≫≫

STANDING LUNGE, LEFT FOOT FORWARD

Stand straight with your feet shoulder-width apart. Step forward with your left foot into a lunge. Bend both knees, lowering your body toward the floor but not letting your right knee touch the floor or your left knee extend over your toes. Rise back into the starting position. Continue to work the same leg for a full 30 seconds.

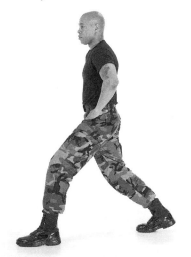
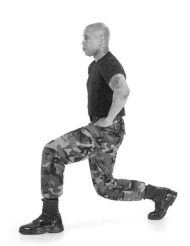

Welcome to Lunging

Lunges tone the thighs and help with balance. They tone your ass and your hips, and you will end up with a very nice, tight hip and thigh area if you do this exercise properly. To get properly toned, you need to work each group of muscles, so it's important to do this exercise equally on both sides of the body.

In my workout I say, "Left lunge first." That's just military: In the Marine Corps we start with the left. We even teach our boxers to stand left foot first. It's a marine tradition and it's one more way that we're unique.

But you need to do right lunges as well, so that you balance out the groups of muscles. Again this is an exercise that works naturally with your own body weight to coach you in perfect balance. You don't need a gym machine for that; you just need a patch of floor.

MARCH ON THE SPOT (2ND GEAR) ≫≫≫≫≫≫≫≫≫≫≫≫≫≫≫≫≫≫≫

STANDING LUNGE, RIGHT FOOT FORWARD

Stand straight with your feet shoulder-width apart. Step forward with your right foot into a lunge. Bend both knees, lowering your body toward the floor but not letting your left knee touch the floor or your right knee extend over your toes. Continue to work the same leg for a full 30 seconds.

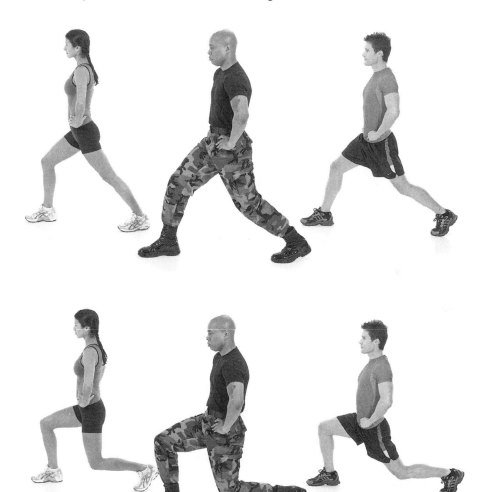

MARCH ON THE SPOT (2ND GEAR) »»»»»»»»»»»»»»»»»»»»»»

SINGLE STANDING CALF RAISE

Stand straight with your hands on your hips. Lift your right foot slightly off the floor and wrap it around the left leg just above the ankle, slightly touching the outside of the left leg. Lift onto the toes of your right foot with a two count and then back down with a two count. Return to standing. Lift your left foot slightly off the floor and wrap it around the right leg just above the ankle, slightly touching the outside of the right leg. Lift onto the toes of your left foot with a two count and then back down with a two count.

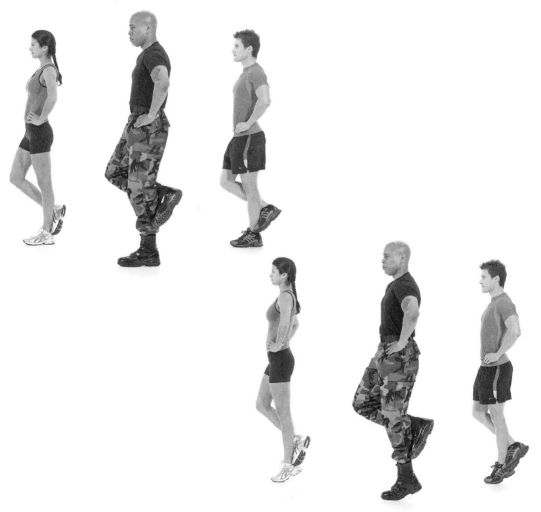

MARCH ON THE SPOT (2ND GEAR) »»»»»»»»»»»»»»»»»»»»»»»»

STEAM ENGINES

Stand with feet shoulder-width apart and place your hands behind your ears. Start by lifting the left foot up, bringing the knee in front of you, at the same time keeping your hands behind your ears while bringing the right elbow down and across to touch the right elbow to the left knee. Then repeat on the opposite side.

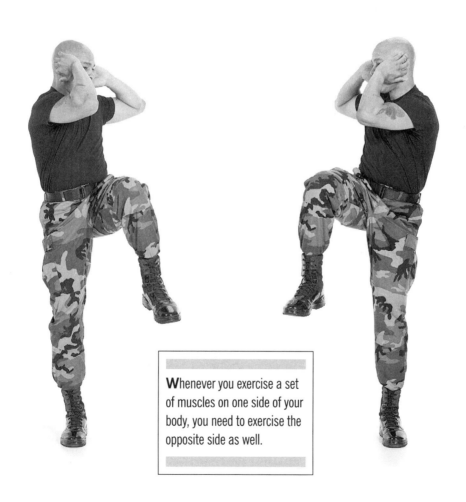

Whenever you exercise a set of muscles on one side of your body, you need to exercise the opposite side as well.

MARCH ON THE SPOT (2ND GEAR) ≫≫≫≫≫≫≫≫≫≫≫≫≫≫≫≫≫≫

CRUNCH

This exercise will be performed with your hands behind your ears, and you should imagine that there is a big healthy apple under your chin. Lie face up on the floor with your knees bent and feet flat on the floor. Contract up for a count of one, bringing shoulder blades off the floor and back down for one repetition.

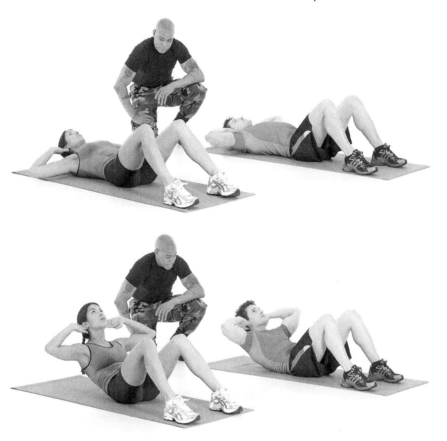

There's a big difference between crunches and sit-ups. Sit-ups are bad for you: They put a strain on your neck and lower back. Watch your head, neck, and hand posture to ensure that it's your abdominal muscles doing the work—NOT your spine.

MARCH ON THE SPOT (2ND GEAR) >>>>>>>>>>>>>>>>>>>>>>>>>>>>>>>>

BODY TWIST WITH KNEES BENT

Lie on your back with your arms extended straight out from your shoulders. Bend your knees and raise your feet. Starting to the left first, you will rotate both knees to the left, then back to center, then to the right, in a controlled motion. Continue rotating for the complete 30 seconds.

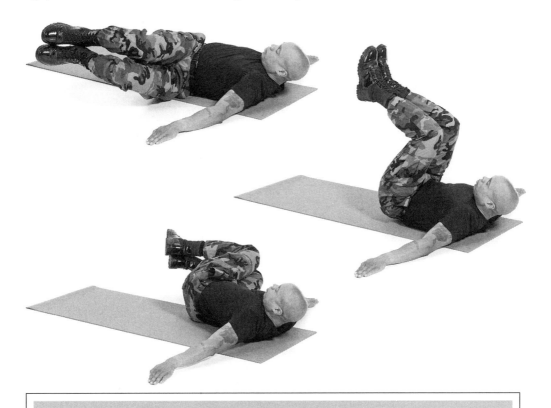

I used to hate these exercises, but you can't do without body twists if you're going to work both your abs and your obliques and get a trim physique and strong, fit core muscles. If your obliques have been neglected, a full body twist can be very difficult, which is why, for this workout, I've given you this easy version.

MARCH ON THE SPOT (2ND GEAR)

LEG LIFTS

Lie on your back with your legs extended and your toes pointing away from you. You may place your hands under your butt for support. Keeping legs and feet together, raise both off the floor straight up until your toes are pointing at the sky above, then back down until feet are about 6 inches above the floor.

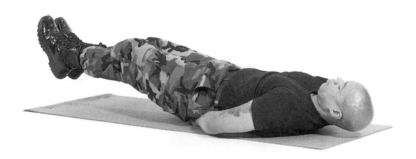

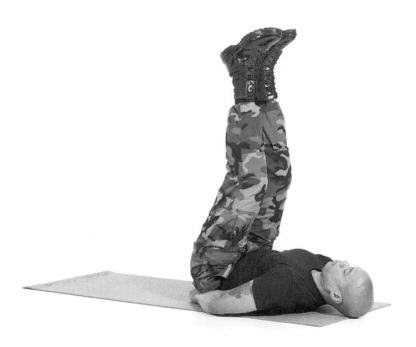

MARCH ON THE SPOT (2ND GEAR) »»»»»»»»»»»»»»»»»»»»»»

FLUTTER KICKS

Lie on your back with your legs extended and your toes pointing away from you. Instead of raising both feet and legs at the same time, you will start with the left first, then alternate with the right, and continue alternating just as if you were swimming.

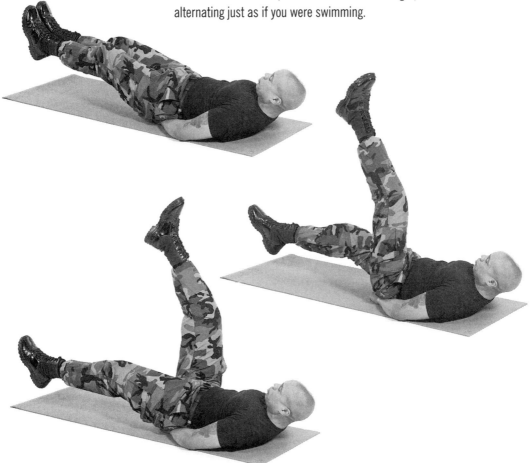

In the marines we did a variation of flutter kicks sitting on the edge of the pool wearing fins. The fins were light at first, but by the time you raised and lowered your legs four hundred times they sure felt heavy. And by the time you got to five hundred, you wanted out.

Cooling down is just as important as warming up to

make sure your body remains in top fighting fitness. If you have a

great workout, and then don't cool down, you're putting yourself at

risk of injury from strains. And you'll be sore the next day, which is

not part of our plan. **So stay smart** and do your

marches and stretches, and then you're still in the fight and

READY TO ROCK.

MARCH ON THE SPOT

Relax and control breathing.

(2ND GEAR) (3 MINUTES)

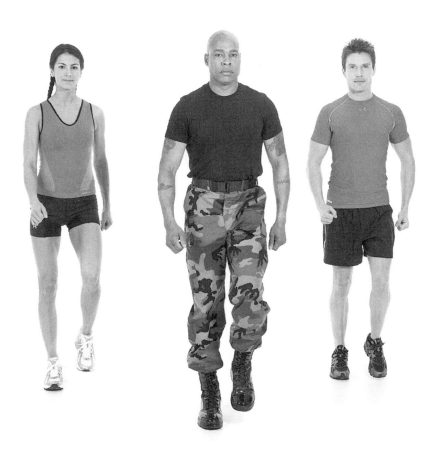

MARCH ON THE SPOT
(1ST GEAR) (3 MINUTES)

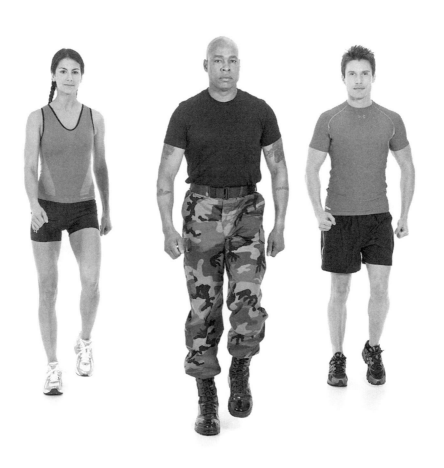

NECK STRETCH

Standing with feet shoulder-width apart, lean your head to the left, stretching the right side. Hold for a count of 20, then switch and repeat.

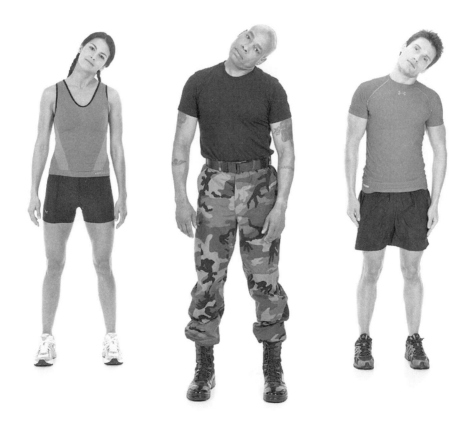

TRICEPS STRETCH

Stand with your feet shoulder-width apart. Bend the left elbow and place your left hand between your shoulder blades. Gently pull the left elbow with the right hand. Hold for a count of 20. Switch arms and repeat.

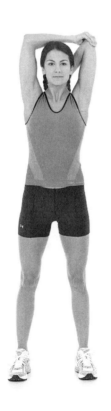
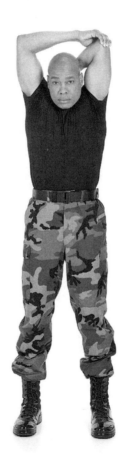
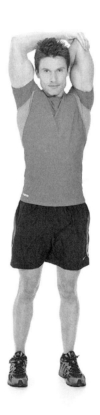

SHOULDER STRETCH

Stand with your feet shoulder-width apart. Bring your left arm across your chest and give a gentle pull with the right hand. Hold for a count of 20. Switch arms and repeat.

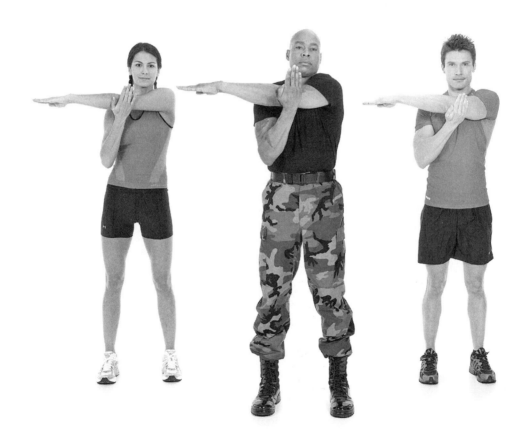

CHEST STRETCH

Stand with your feet shoulder-width apart. Clasp hands together behind the lower back with palms facing up. Pull arms toward the sky and hold for a count of 20.

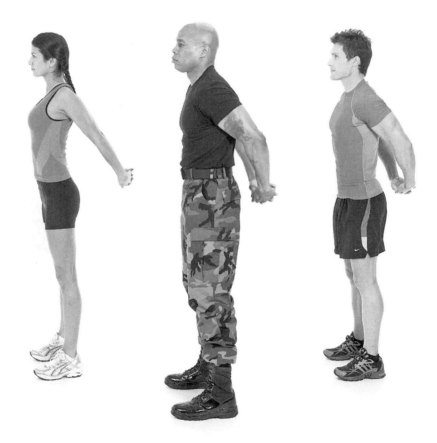

UPPER BACK STRETCH

Stand with your feet shoulder-width apart. Extend your arms in front of you at shoulder height with hands clasped and palms facing away from you. Push arms forward, rounding upper back while bending your knees slightly. Hold for a count of 20.

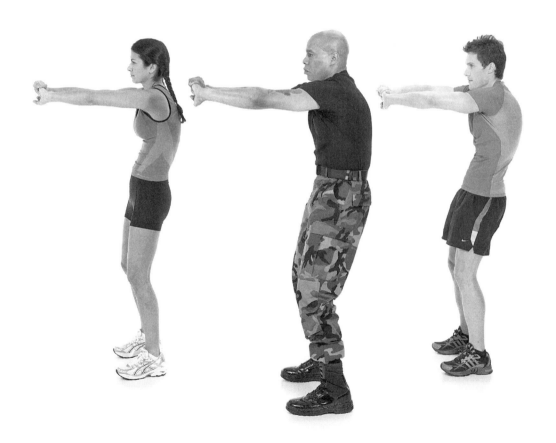

HAMSTRING STRETCH

Lie on your back. Bring your left knee toward your chest, grasping the left leg below the knee. The right knee should be slightly bent and the right foot remains on the floor. Hold for a count of 20. Switch legs and repeat.

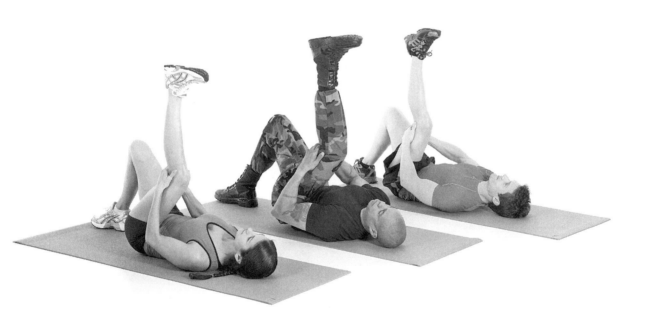

CALF STRETCH

Stand with your feet shoulder-width apart. Place your right foot in front of you, keeping both feet pointing forward and both heels on the floor. Bend the right knee slightly as you feel the stretch in the left calf. Hold for a count of 20. Switch legs and repeat.

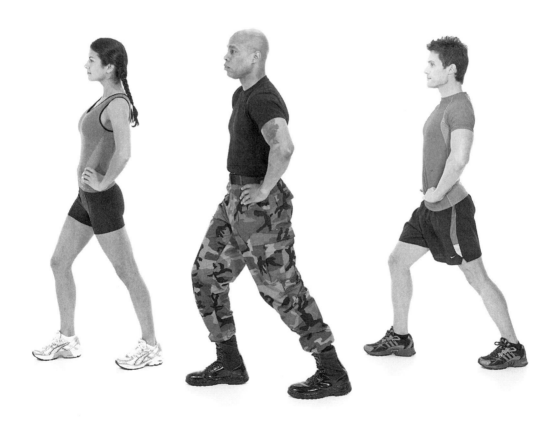

GROIN STRETCH

Sitting with both knees bent and bottoms of the feet together, grasp the feet and push your knees, with your elbows toward the floor. Hold for a count of 20.

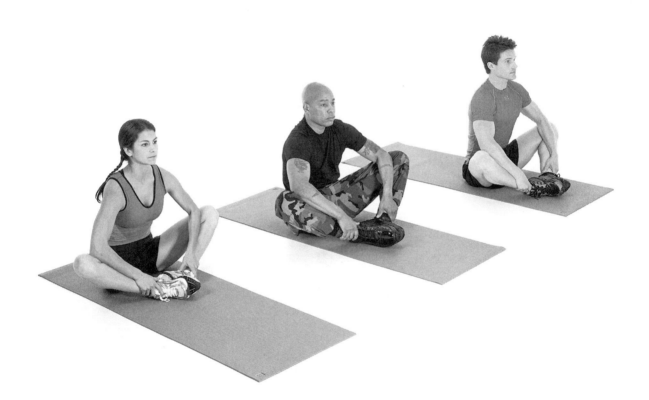

QUAD STRETCH

Lie on the floor on your right side. Grab the left ankle with the left hand and pull the left knee straight back. Hold for a count of 20. Switch legs and repeat.

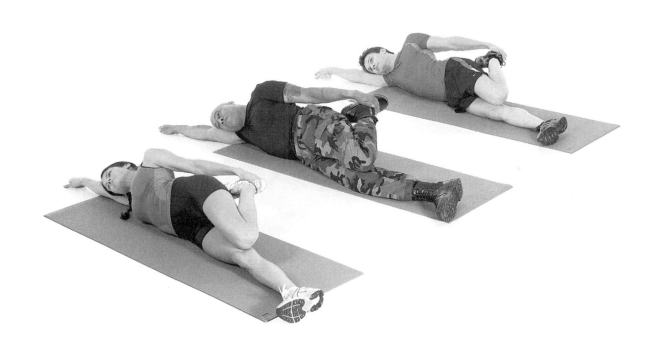

LOW BACK STRETCH

Lie on your back. Bring the left knee toward your chest with your right leg remaining on the floor. Hold for a count of 20. Switch legs and repeat.

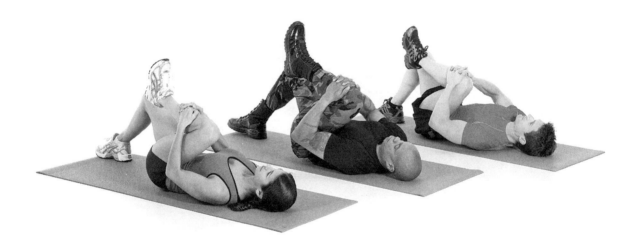

STAGE TWO:
NOW YOU ARE IN THE FIGHT

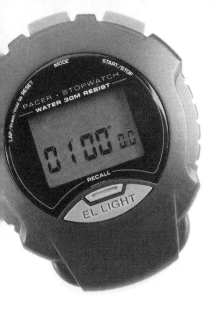

You've gotten off your butt, you've moved out of your comfort zone, and now **you're definitely in the fight against obesity.** From here we take initials because we don't have time to take names.

After six weeks of eating healthily and doing Stage One four times a week, 30 minutes at a time, you've started to breathe easier, you've come out of your comfort zone, and **now it's time to move on to the bigger, better things in life.** Take a bow because your body will have changed; it's stronger and fitter. From here on out, it's just going to get better.

It's not going to be easy, but we've got to do it because it's the way forward. You know that. So it will get better, and you must hang in there and **stay in the fight.**

You've got to give yourself more to do and keep your body surprised so that it doesn't get used to always doing the same thing. That's why we change the workout every six weeks.

Because you've gotten fitter and leaner, we need to keep you working, so we double the time to do each exercise, from 30 seconds to **1 minute. And the exercises get tougher too.**

But as usual, grasshoppers, we start off with the warm-up.

MARCH ON THE SPOT
(1 MINUTE)

Your feet are shoulder-width apart, and your hands are at your sides as you begin to pick your feet up ankle high and pump arms simultaneously.

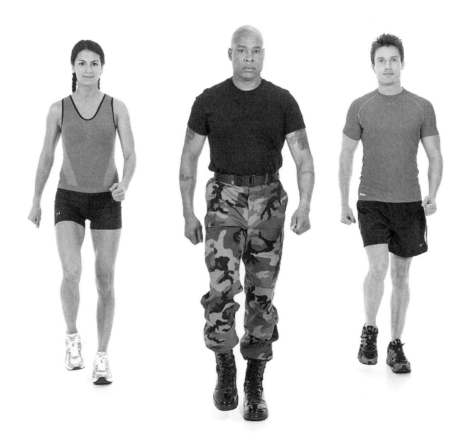

>>>>>> # STEAM ENGINES
(1 MINUTE)

Feet are shoulder-width apart and hands are behind your ears. Start by lifting the left foot up, bringing the knee in front of you, at the same time keeping the hands behind the ears, touching the right elbow to the left knee. Then repeat on the opposite side. >>>>>>

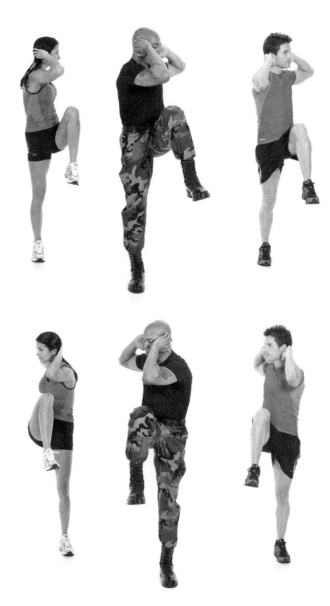

SIDE STRADDLE HOPS
(1 MINUTE)

Start with the feet together and your hands at your sides. Jump outward and land with both feet wider than shoulder-width apart while swinging your arms outward and up until your hands meet over your head. Reverse these actions as you jump back to the starting position.

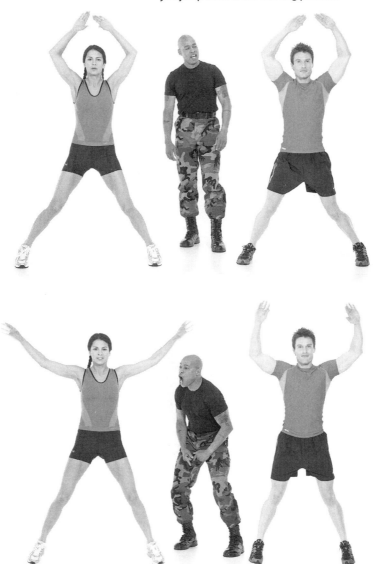

NECK STRETCH

Standing with feet shoulder-width apart, lean your head to the left, stretching the right side. Hold for a count of 10, switch, and repeat.

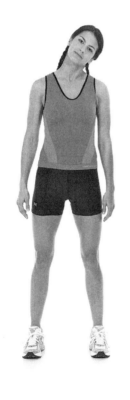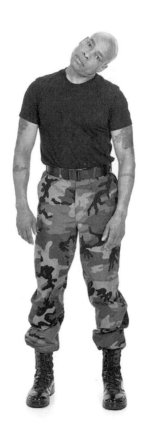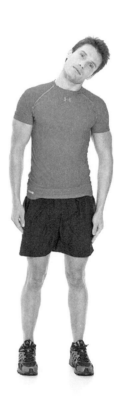

TRICEPS STRETCH

Stand with your feet shoulder-width apart. Bend the left elbow and place your left hand between your shoulder blades. Gently pull the left elbow with the right hand. Hold for a count of 10. Switch arms and repeat.

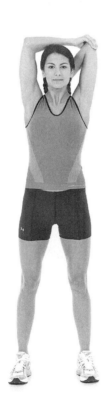
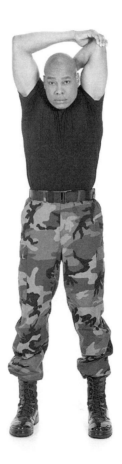
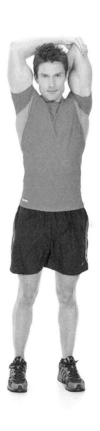

SHOULDER STRETCH

Stand with your feet shoulder-width apart. Bring your left arm across your chest and give it a gentle pull with the right hand. Hold for a count of 10. Switch arms and repeat.

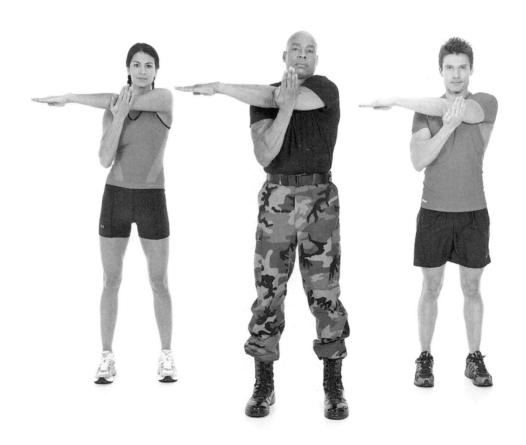

CHEST STRETCH

Stand with your feet shoulder-width apart. Clasp hands together behind the lower back with palms facing up. Pull arms toward the sky and hold for a count of 10.

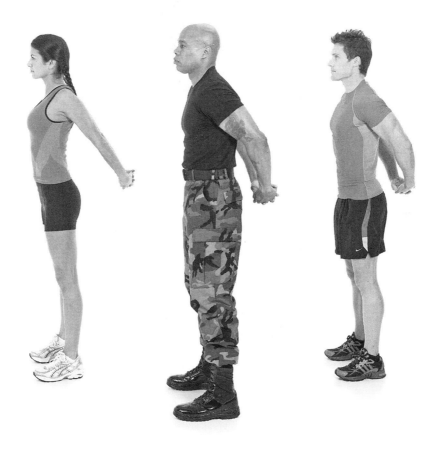

UPPER BACK STRETCH

Stand with your feet shoulder-width apart. Extend your arms in front of you at shoulder height with hands clasped and palms facing away from you. Push arms forward, rounding upper back while bending your knees slightly. Hold for a count of 10.

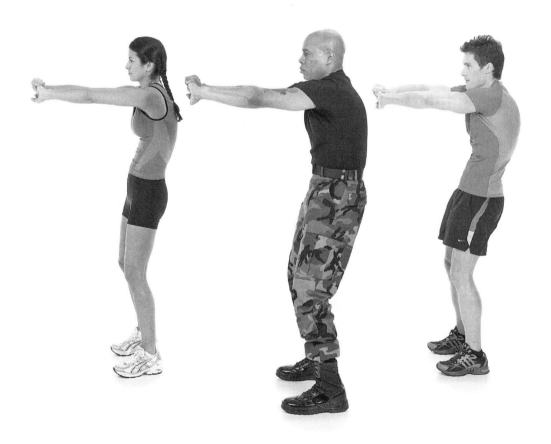

HAMSTRING STRETCH

Lie on your back. Bring your left knee toward your chest, grasping the left leg below the knee. The right knee should be slightly bent, and the right foot remains on the floor. Hold for a count of 10. Switch legs and repeat.

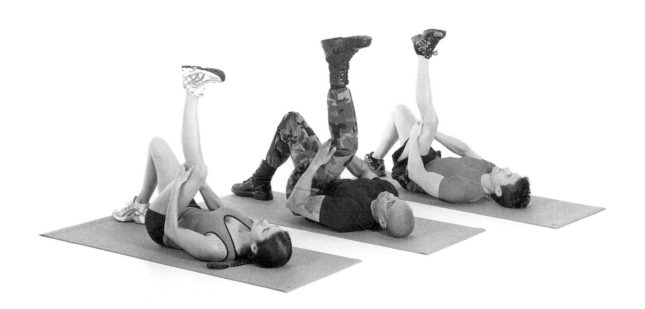

CALF STRETCH

Stand with your feet shoulder-width apart. Place your right foot in front of you, keeping both feet pointing forward and both heels on the floor. Bend the right knee slightly as you feel the stretch in the left calf. Hold for a count of 10. Switch legs and repeat.

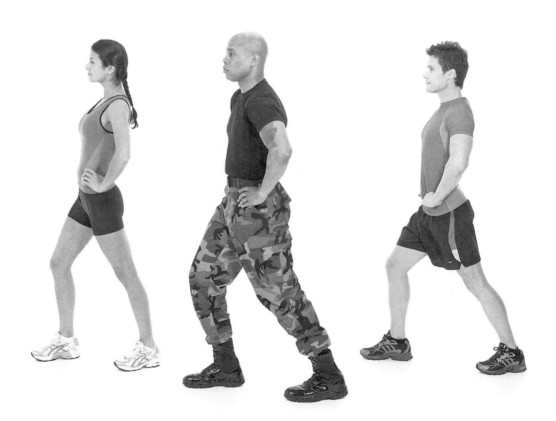

>>>>>> # GROIN STRETCH
Sitting with both knees bent and bottoms of the feet together, grasp the feet and push your knees with your elbows toward the floor. Hold for a count of 10. >>>>>>

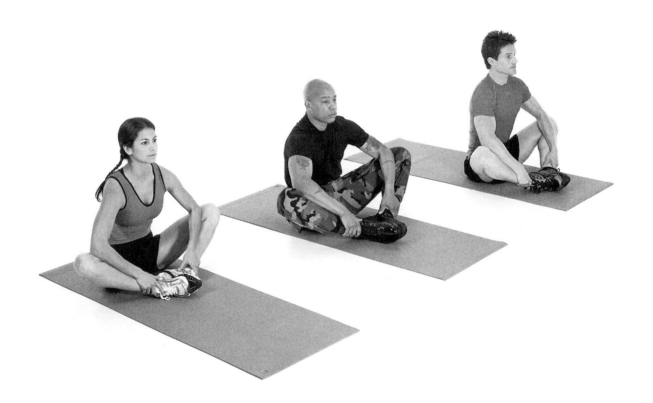

QUAD STRETCH

Lie on the floor on your right side. Grab the left ankle with the left hand and pull the left knee straight back. Hold for a count of 10. Switch legs and repeat.

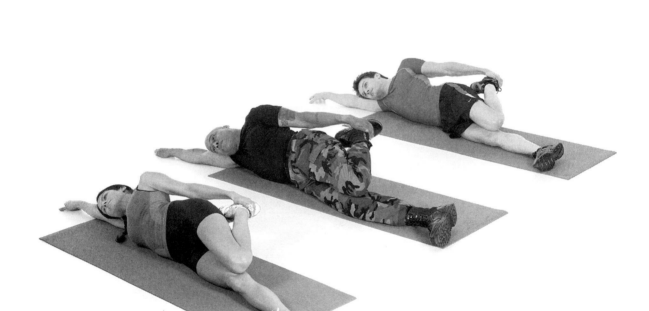

LOW BACK STRETCH

Lie on your back. Bring the left knee toward your chest, with your right leg remaining on the floor. Hold for a count of 10. Switch legs and repeat.

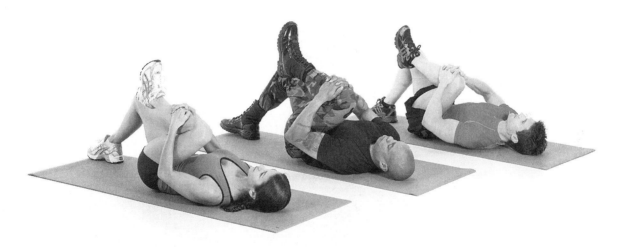

MARCH ON THE SPOT
(1ST GEAR)

Feet are shoulder-width apart, hands are at your sides, and you begin to pick your feet up ankle high and pump arms simultaneously.

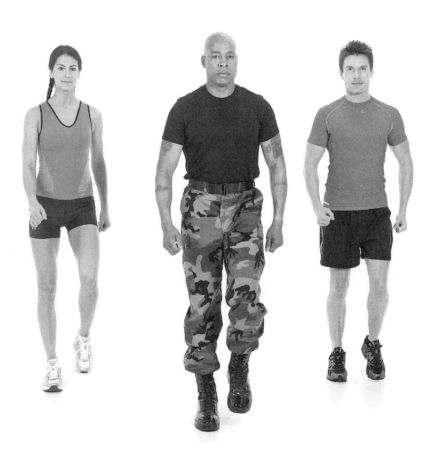

SIDE STRADDLE HOP

Start with your feet together and your hands at your sides. Jump outward and land with both feet wider than shoulder-width apart while swinging your arms outward and up until your hands meet over your head. Reverse these actions as you jump back to the starting position.

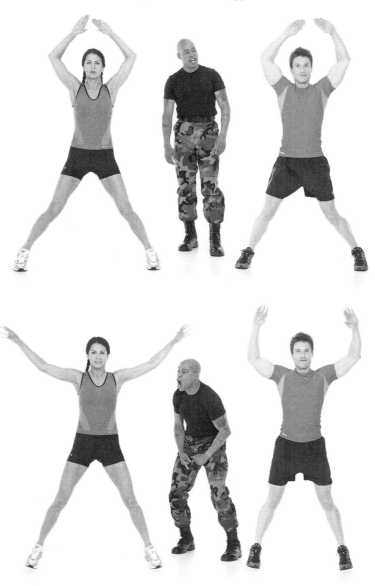

MARCH ON THE SPOT (1 MINUTE, 1ST GEAR)

SCISSOR JACK

Similar to cross-country skiing but without the ski poles and skis.

Scissor jack is about sliding, and you should take it slow and do it for the full 1 minute.

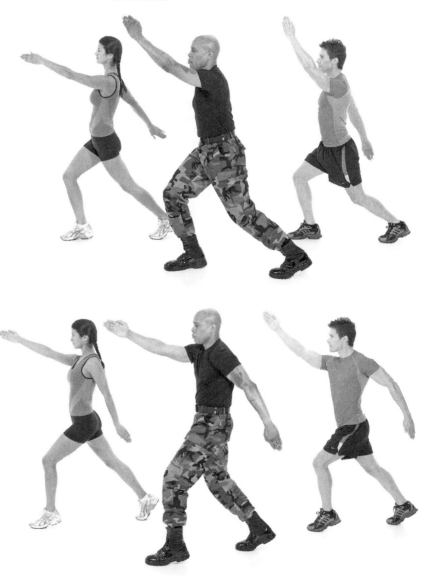

MARCH ON THE SPOT (1ST GEAR) ⟫⟫⟫⟫⟫⟫⟫⟫⟫⟫⟫⟫⟫⟫⟫⟫⟫⟫⟫⟫

HALF JACK

This starts in the same position as the side straddle hop. Spread your feet apart, but instead of your hands going above your head, your hands and arms will come only halfway up until they are about shoulder height, with palms facing the floor.

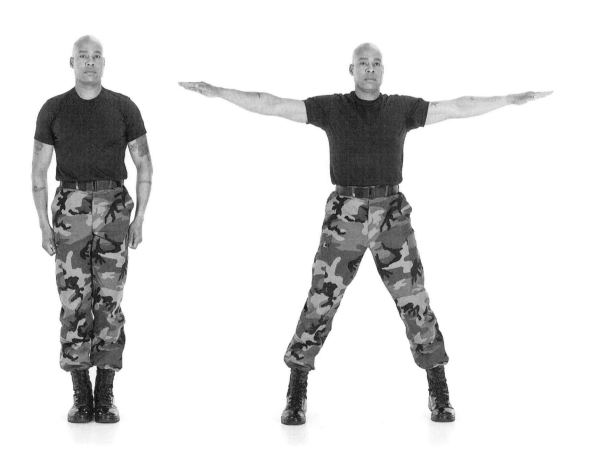

MARCH ON THE SPOT (1ST GEAR) »»»»»»»»»»»»»»»»»»»»»

ARM ROTATIONS TO SIDE LATERAL FORWARD

Stand with your feet shoulder-width apart. Raise your arms until they are shoulder height, straight out to your sides, with palms facing downward. Rotate in small circles forward.

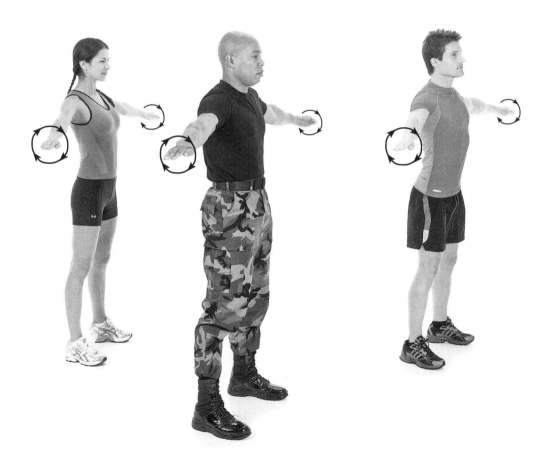

ARM ROTATIONS, FRONT

Here your arms and hands are in front of your body at shoulder height and shoulder width, with the palms of your hands facing each other. Rotate your arms outward, making small circles.

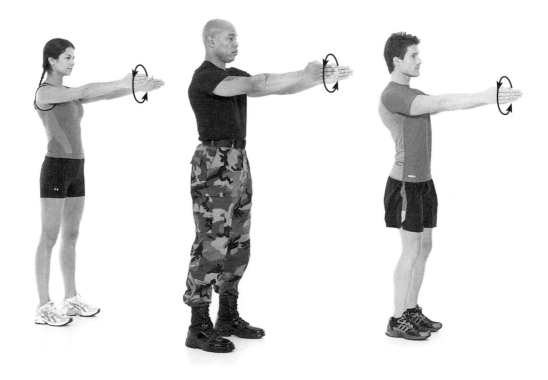

SIDE STRADDLE HOP
(2ND GEAR)

Start with your feet together and your hands at your side. Jump outward and land with both feet wider than shoulder-width apart while swinging your arms outward and up until your hands meet over your head. Reverse these actions as you jump back to the starting position.

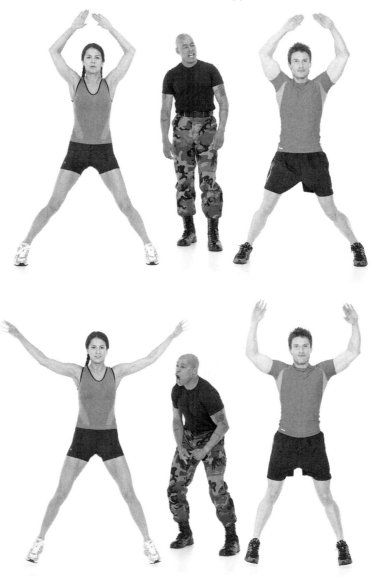

Harvey's Favorite Workout Music

I have more than 7,000 songs on my iPod, so you can pretty much make the assumption that I love music. When I'm doing cardio or am out on runs, I usually go back to my Chicago roots and listen to house music, acid jazz (Gilles Peterson and Gnarls Barkley really rock) or some garage music.

When I'm lifting weights I listen to a little bit of everything from Nickelback and Hinder to Prince and Seal. I am also a TRUE FAN of jazz. In fact my car stays on the Jazz Café on Sirius unless I'm on my way to the gym, then I jam to the Beat or Strobe. Satellite radio is the best kept secret for music lovers. When I'm at home relaxing I normally just relax on my deck with the iPod and listen to jazz. I have a wooded area behind my house so I see all sorts of creatures of nature relaxing as well and we sort of look at each other and mind our own business. I connect my speakers to the iPod so they may be enjoying the music as well. Below are some of my favorite artists.

JAZZ/EASY LISTENING

John Mayer	Boney James	Herbie Hancock
Corinne Bailey Rae	Wayman Tisdale	Jamie Cullum
Michael Bublé	Chuck Loeb	Kirk Whalum
Gerald Levert	Kenny G	Pat Metheny
India.Arie	Veronica Martell (love her to death)	Rick Braun
Heather Headley	Al Jarreau	Katie Melua
Robin Thicke	Anita Baker	Sade
Norah Jones	Chris Botti	James Blunt
Walter Beasle	Diana Krall	

. . . just to name a few. I love my music, as you can see.

WORKOUT MUSIC

Nickelback	Hinder	U2
Daughtry	Joss Stone	Jamiroquai
Gwen Stefani	Seal	house music
The Fray	Gilles Peterson	
Prince	Gnarls Barkley	

PUSH-UPS: 3 DOWN, 1 UP

The push-ups here will be performed with hands shoulder-width apart and started in the up position. You will go down for three counts at three different levels, and at the three count your chest is about 2 inches off the floor. You will then go back up to starting position in one count. This completes one repetition of the exercise. Continue this sequence.

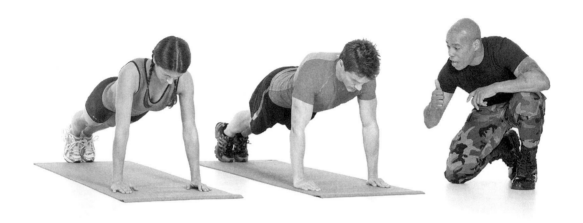

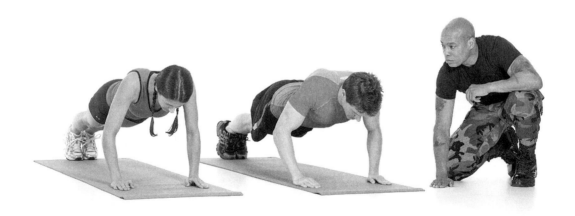

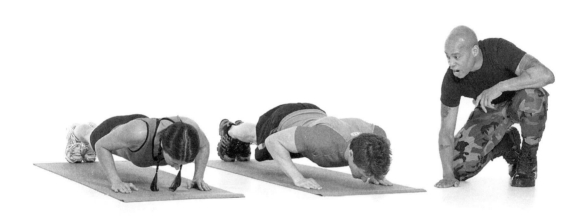

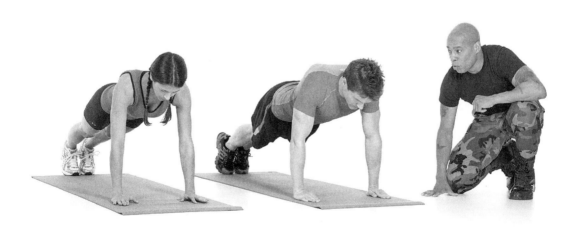

SIDE STRADDLE HOP (2ND GEAR)

DIAMOND PUSH-UPS: 2 DOWN, 2 UP

Lie on your stomach. Place your hands under your chest with the index fingers of each hand and both thumbs touching, forming the shape of a diamond. All other fingers are extended. You will perform the exercise just as you would a normal push-up with the exception of going down in two counts and coming up in two.

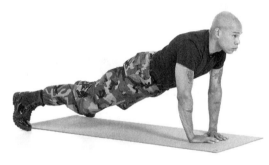
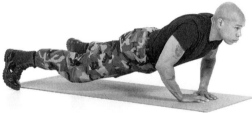
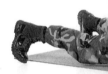

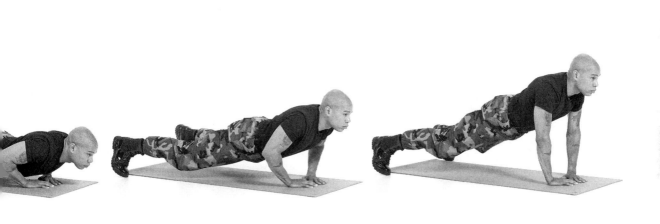

SIDE STRADDLE HOP (2ND GEAR) ≫≫≫≫≫≫≫≫≫≫≫≫≫≫≫≫≫≫≫≫≫≫≫

WIDE PUSH-UPS: 2 DOWN, 2 UP

Lie on your stomach. Place your hands slightly wider than shoulder-width apart, with your fingers extended and each thumb joined along the hand. You will go down in two counts, and at the second count your chest will be about 2 inches off the deck. You will push up in two separate counts with the second count bringing you back to the original starting position.

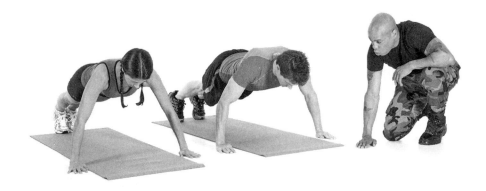

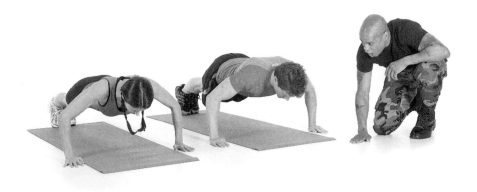

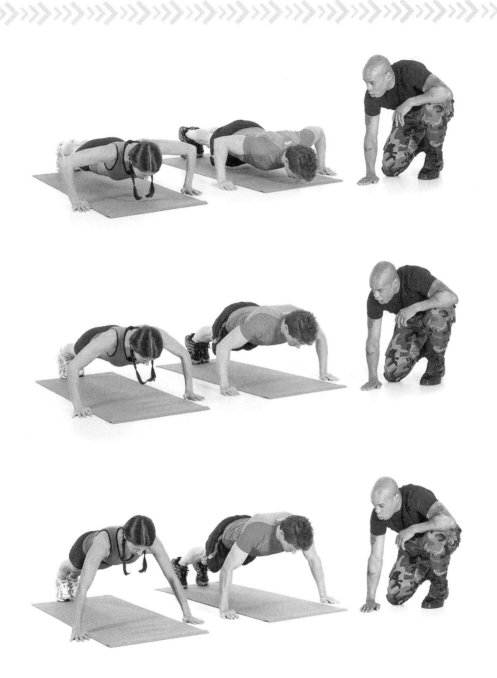

SIDE STRADDLE HOP (2ND GEAR) >>>>>>>>>>>>>>>>>>>>>>>>>>>>>>>

PUSH-UPS: 1 DOWN, 3 UP

Here push-ups will be performed with one count down until your chest is about 2 inches off the floor and pushing up in three counts until you are in the starting position at count three.

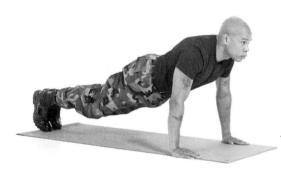
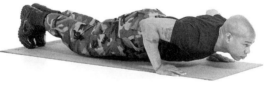
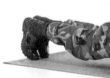

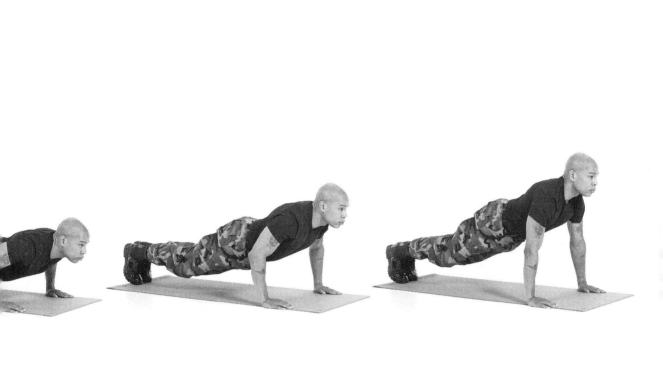

SIDE STRADDLE HOP (3RD GEAR) >>>>>>>>>>>>>>>>>>>>>>>>>>>>>>>>>>>>>>>

SQUATS WITH CALF RAISE: 2 DOWN, 1 UP WITH CALF RAISE

Stand with your feet shoulder-width apart. Extend your arms in front of the body at shoulder height. Squat down for two counts by bending the knees as you lower with each count until the second count has your thighs parallel to the floor. Rise up in one count. Add another count as you rise up on your toes, performing a calf raise. Return to the starting position.

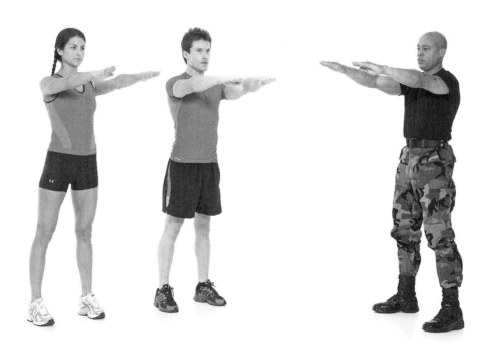

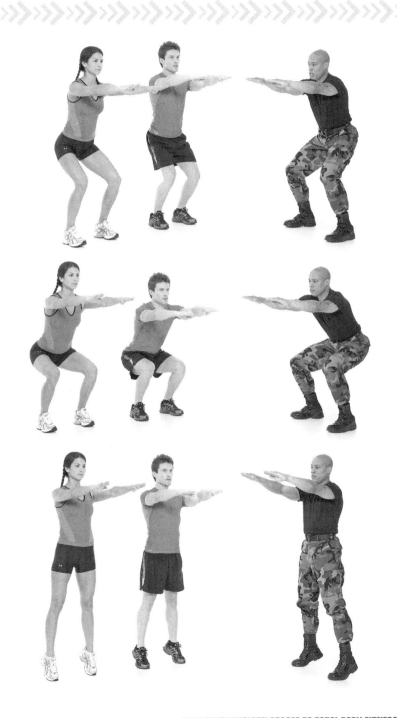

SIDE STRADDLE HOP (3RD GEAR) >>>>>>>>>>>>>>>>>>>>>>>>>

4-COUNT BEAT BOOTS: 3 DOWN, 1 UP

Stand with your feet shoulder-width apart. Extend your arms in front of the body at shoulder height. Squat down for three counts by bending the knees a little more at each level and keeping your belly button pulled in and your weight on your heels. On the third count, lower your hands to your sides and reach around and tap your ankles. Once ankles are tapped, you will stand completely up in one count while raising your arms so that they are again extended in front of you at shoulder height, completing one repetition of the exercise.

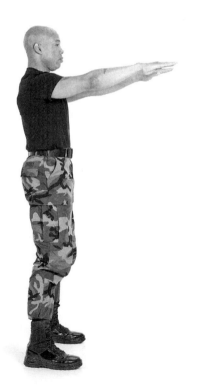
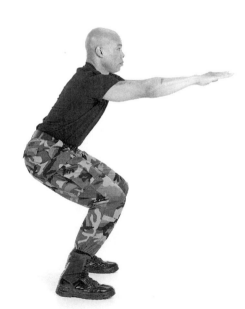

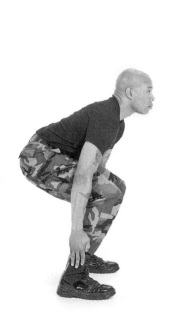
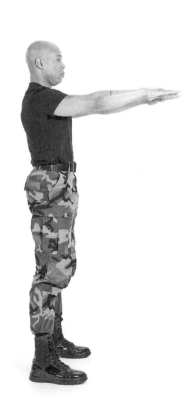

SIDE STRADDLE HOP (3RD GEAR) >>>>>>>>>>>>>>>>>>>>>>>>>>>>
ALTERNATING FORWARD LUNGES

Here the lunges will alternate instead of working one leg at a time. Stand straight with your feet shoulder-width apart. Step forward with your left foot into a lunge. Bend both knees, lowering your body toward the floor but not letting your right knee touch the floor or your left knee extend over the toes. Rise back up into the starting position. Switch sides and repeat.

You've done the first stage of lunges, so now you've got better balance. When you alternate lunges each time, you see how good your balance is, and that helps you work a little more and squeeze that core a bit more.

And now we're in a new fight and we're up to 3rd gear, so it's time to start jogging on the spot to keep that cardio level up and keep burning those calories.

The pain is only going to be temporary, but the pride and respect you will have once it's all said and done will be forever, so suck it up and enjoy the new fab body you are going to get in the end.

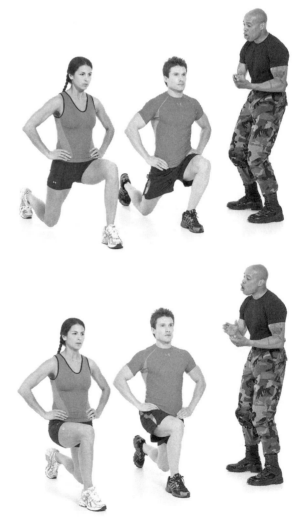

JOG ON THE SPOT
(3RD GEAR)

Start running in place and gradually increase speed as if you are shifting gears in a car and get into 3rd gear.

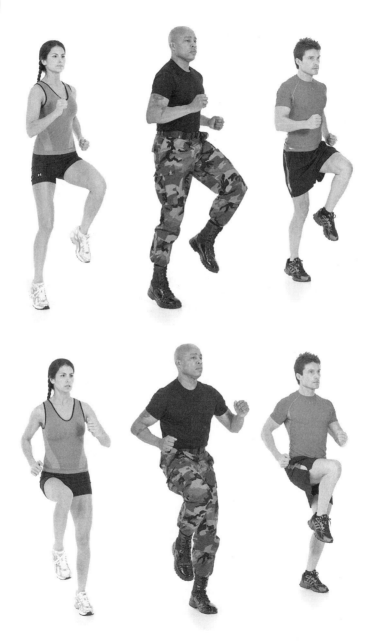

4-COUNT CRUNCHES: 2 UP, 2 DOWN

Lie face up on the floor with your knees bent and your feet flat on the floor. Place your hands behind your ears and imagine that there is a big healthy apple under your chin. Contract up for a count of two, bringing your shoulder blades off the floor in the first count and raising into the crunch on the second count. Then back down to the floor on two counts for one repetition.

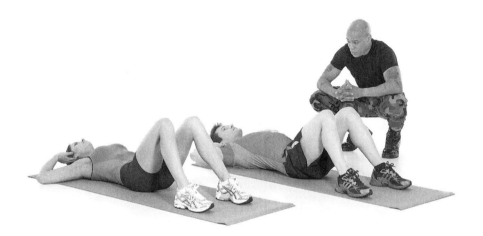

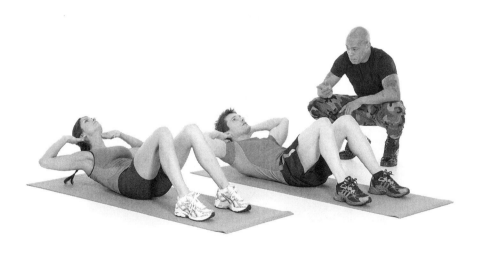

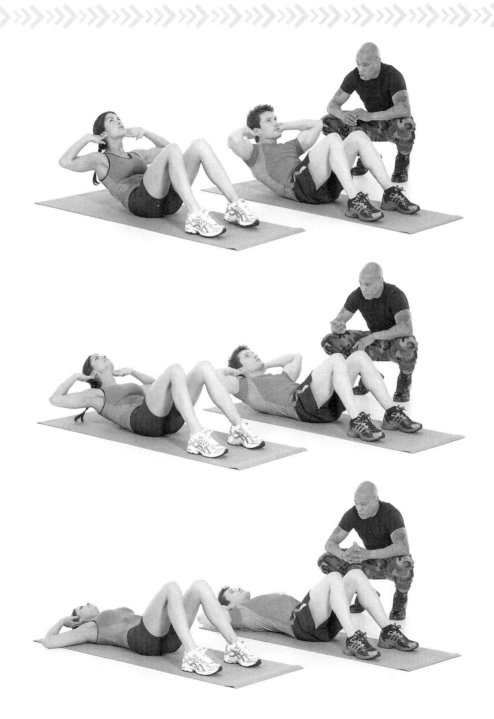

JOG ON THE SPOT (3RD GEAR) »»»»»»»»»»»»»»»»»»»»»»

4-COUNT LEG LIFTS

Lie on your back with your legs extended, raising your feet 6 inches off the floor, with your toes pointing away from you. You may place your hands under your butt for support. Raise your feet up for a count of two, ending with your feet pointing toward the sky and legs at a 90-degree angle, then lower your legs down in two counts until the feet are 6 inches off the floor again.

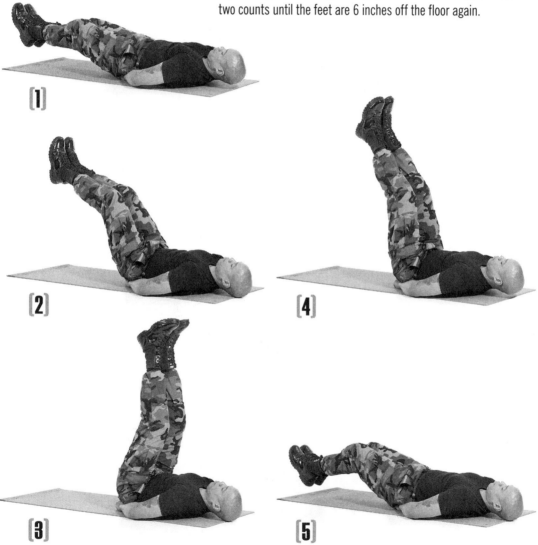

[1]

[2]

[3]

[4]

[5]

JOG ON THE SPOT (3RD GEAR) »»»»»»»»»»»»»»»»»»»»

FLUTTER KICKS

Lie on your back with your legs extended, raising your feet 6 inches off the floor, with your toes pointing away from you. You may place your hands under your butt for support. Start with your left leg and then alternate with the right as if you were swimming. Your feet should never touch the floor.

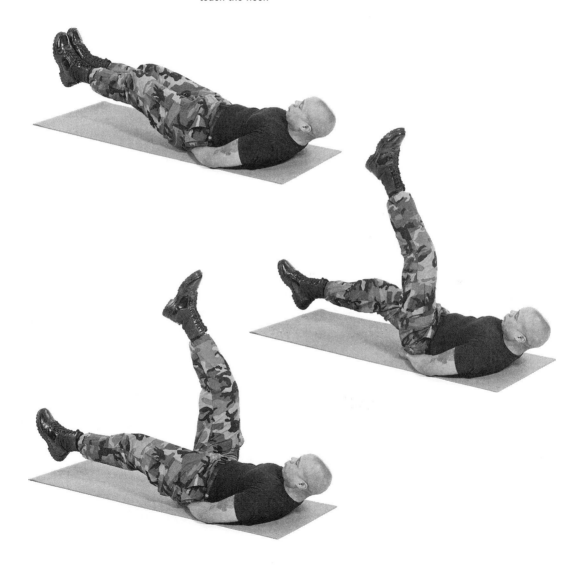

JOG ON THE SPOT (3RD GEAR) »»»»»»»»»»»»»»»»»»»»

4-COUNT HELLO SUNSHINES

Lie on your back with your legs extended, raising your feet 6 inches off the floor, with your toes pointing away from you. On four counts you will start to separate your feet, spreading your legs apart and keeping your feet 6 inches off the floor throughout the whole exercise. After the fourth count, bring feet back together in one motion.

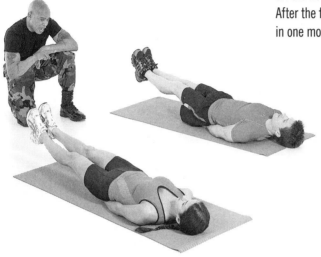

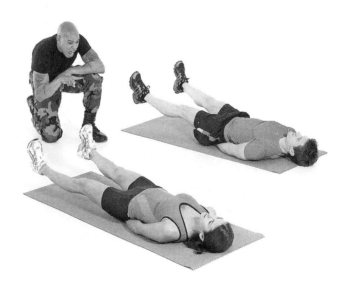

I normally call these exercises Hello Dollies, but for this book I've changed the name to Hello Sunshines, to encourage people to do them in the morning when the sun comes up. It's just a funny thing that keeps you laughing while you're working out. Hello Sunshine is a move I used at Wal-Mart supermarkets when they had me lead a Harvey Walden workout for their staff. That time I called it Hello Tropicana. People went away laughing and they'd had a good workout as well!

JOG ON THE SPOT (3RD GEAR) ≫≫≫≫≫≫≫≫≫≫≫≫≫≫

BODY TWISTS WITH LEGS STRAIGHT

Lie on your back with your arms extended straight out from your shoulders. Legs will be straight up at a 90-degree angle, with the bottom of your feet facing straight up to the sky. Starting to the left, rotate both feet to the left, then back to center, then to the right, in a controlled motion. Continue rotating for the full 1 minute.

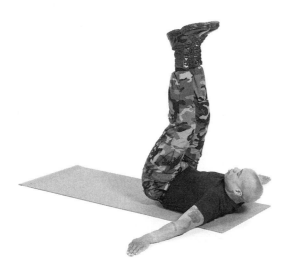
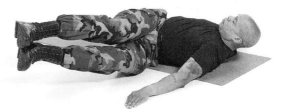

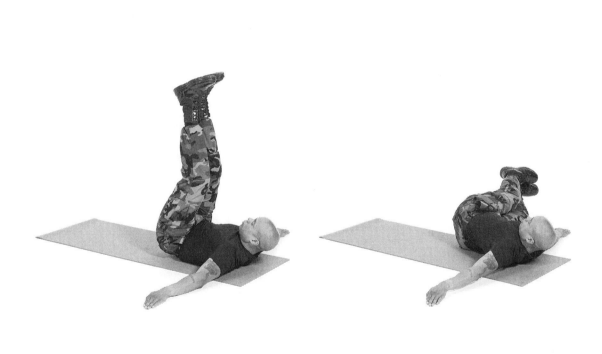

JOG ON THE SPOT (3RD GEAR) »»»»»»»»»»»»»»»»»»

GRASSHOPPER HARVEY BUILDERS WITH ARM ROTATIONS

Stand straight with your feet together and your arms extended to your sides at shoulder height. Make big circles forward for 15 rotations. Now make 15 rotations backward. Immediately after the arm rotations, squat all the way down, touching the floor with your hands on the outside of your feet. Kick both feet out behind you, placing you in a push-up position. You will now perform one regular push-up, then kick your feet back into the squat position and stand up. After the arm rotations, the first count is the squat, second count is the feet kicking back, third count is the down feet coming back in, placing you in squat position, with hands on the outside of each foot, and the fourth count will be you standing up into the starting position for one repetition. Keep performing this sequence for the complete minute.

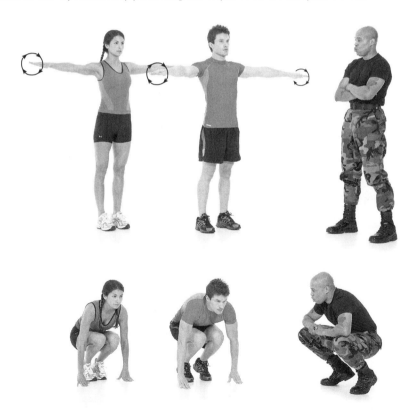

When I was at drill-instructor school, a three-month school that sends you back to boot camp, there was an exercise the instructors called the Jack Webb, (the actor who played Joe Friday on *Dragnet*), which used to really kick my ass. This right here is my version of what the Jack Webb was. It was the kind of twist that made you want to throw something in the air and kick ass at the end and you were in the fight.

Drill-instructor school was incredibly hard. Who wants to go to boot camp again? We were all staff sergeants, and man, we didn't want to do this bullshit, we wanted to kill recruits with these exercises. You go as senior staff non-commissioned officers, get freakin' humiliated, beat down, wore the hell out, and it's tough. It's worse than going to doggone SEAR (survival training) school, really.

I had a class of maybe 30, and this exercise, man, it burned your arms. We had to sit there and do these, and the way we did them was, you do one, then one push-up, two, two-push-ups, and you'd think, *Oh, God, it's killing me,* and you couldn't do anything about it.

So I came up with something similar to the Jack Webb that we can accomplish here without all that pain.

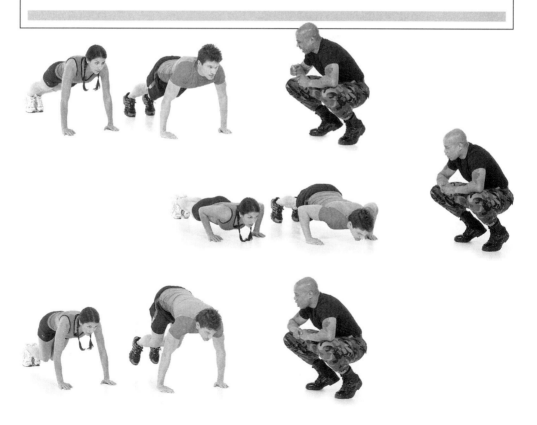

JOG ON THE SPOT (2ND GEAR) (3 MINUTES)

JOG ON THE SPOT (1ST GEAR) (3 MINUTES)

MARCH ON THE SPOT (3 MINUTES)

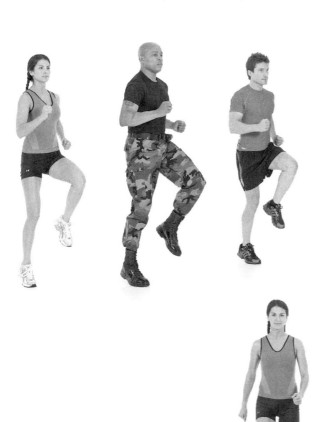

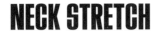

NECK STRETCH

Standing with feet shoulder-width apart, lean your head to the left, stretching the right side. Hold for a count of 10, switch, and repeat.

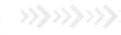

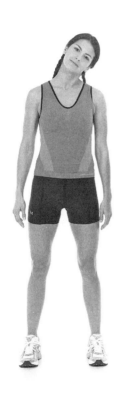

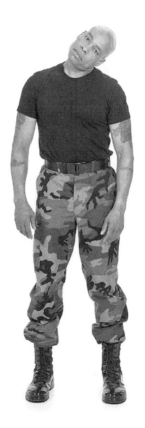

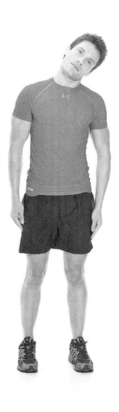

TRICEPS STRETCH

Stand with your feet shoulder-width apart. Bend the left elbow and place your left hand between your shoulder blades. Gently pull the left elbow with the right hand. Hold for a count of 10. Switch arms and repeat.

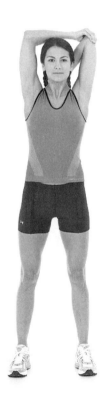
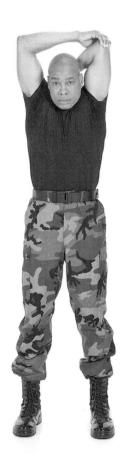
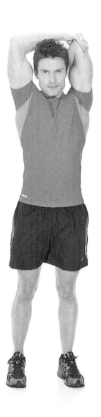

SHOULDER STRETCH

Stand with your feet shoulder-width apart. Bring your left arm across your chest and give it a gentle pull with the right hand. Hold for a count of 10. Switch arms and repeat.

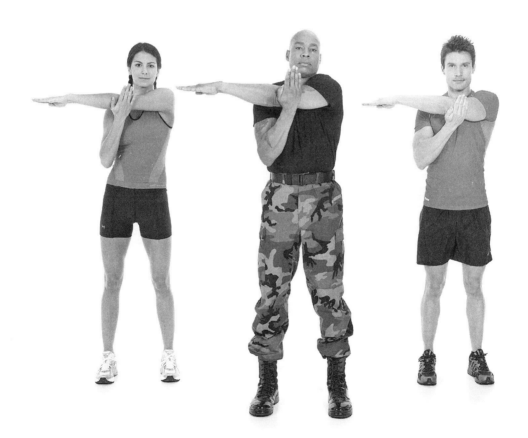

CHEST STRETCH

Stand with your feet shoulder-width apart. Clasp your hands together behind your lower back with the palms facing up. Pull your arms toward the sky and hold for a count of 10.

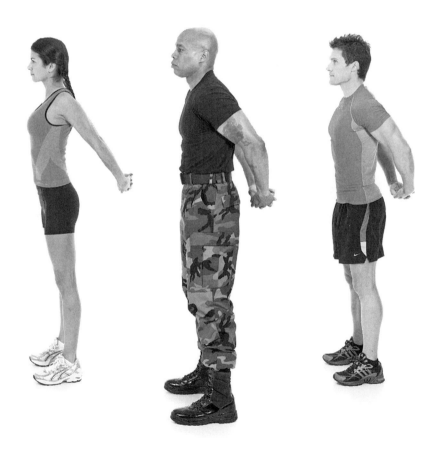

UPPER BACK STRETCH

Stand with your feet shoulder-width apart. Extend your arms in front of you at shoulder height with hands clasped and palms facing away from you. Push your arms forward, rounding your upper back while bending your knees slightly. Hold for a count of 10.

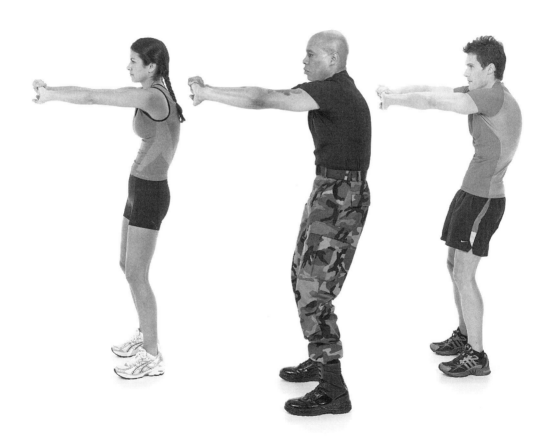

HAMSTRING STRETCH

Lie on your back. Bring your left knee toward your chest, grasping the left leg below the knee. The right knee should be slightly bent and the right foot remains on the floor. Hold for a count of 10. Switch legs and repeat.

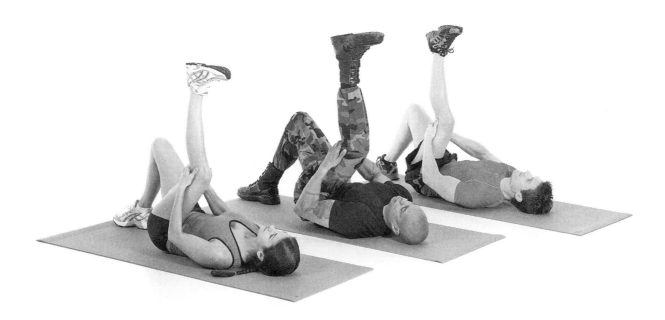

CALF STRETCH

Stand with your feet shoulder-width apart. Place your right foot in front of you, keeping both feet pointing forward and both heels on the floor. Bend the right knee slightly as you feel the stretch in the left calf. Hold for a count of 10. Switch legs and repeat.

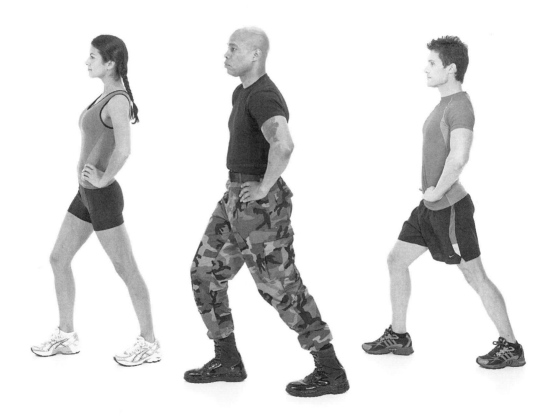

GROIN STRETCH

Sitting with both knees bent and bottoms of the feet together, grasp the feet and push your knees, with your elbows toward the floor. Hold for a count of 10.

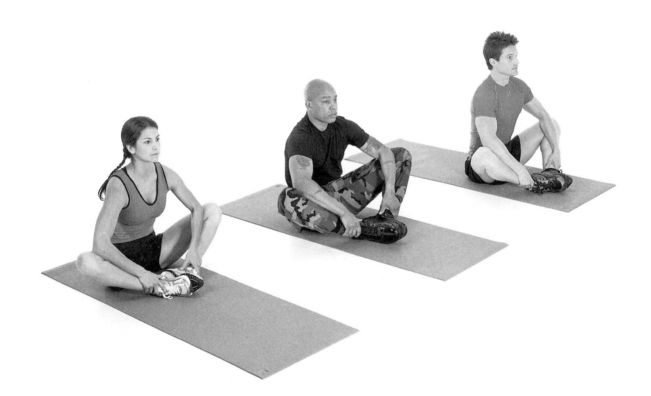

QUAD STRETCH

Lie on the floor on your right side. Grab the left ankle with the left hand and pull the left knee straight back. Hold for a count of 10. Switch legs and repeat.

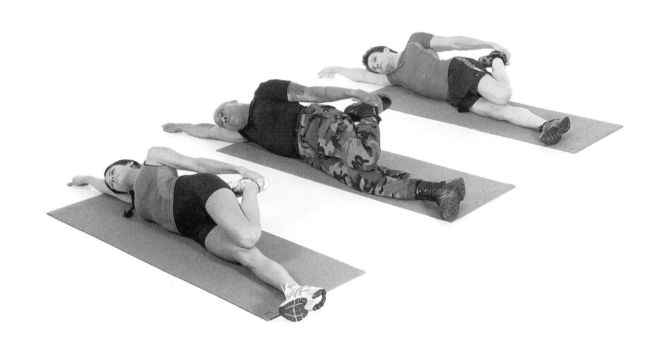

LOW BACK STRETCH

Lie on your back. Bring the left knee toward your chest, with your right leg remaining on the floor. Hold for a count of 10. Switch legs and repeat.

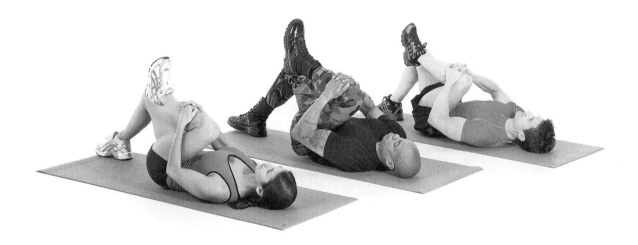

STAGE THREE:
OOH RAH!
YOU'RE A STUD
OR STUDETTE

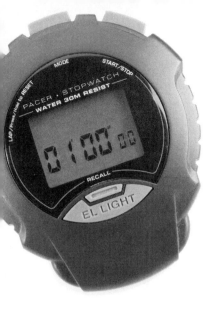

You are a stud now, **so dig deep,** grasshopper, »»»»»

and **stay in the fight** with me. This stage is

much harder, but it will take you where you want to go.

Remember to warm up, and

notice that in this stage you won't have to jog on the spot until you

complete a series of exercises first.

It's your life, your world,

so take control and let's

WIN THIS
BATTLE.

MARCH ON THE SPOT
(1 MINUTE)

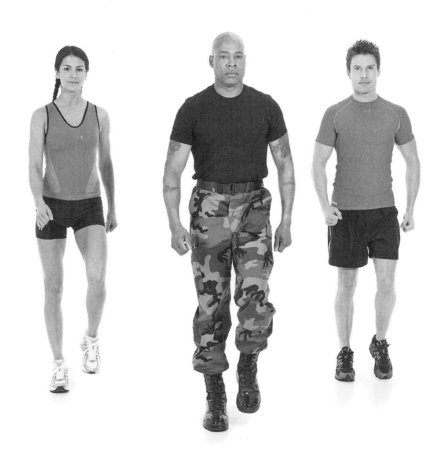

STEAM ENGINES
(1 MINUTE)

Feet are shoulder-width apart and hands are behind your ears. Start by lifting the left foot up, bringing the knee in front of you and at the same time keeping the hands behind the ears, touching the right elbow to the left knee. Then repeat on the opposite side.

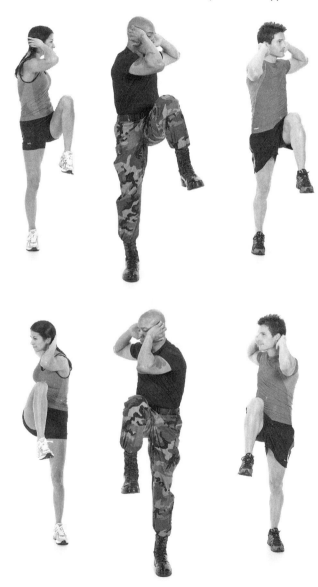

SIDE STRADDLE HOP
(1 MINUTE)

Start with your feet together and your hands at your sides. Jump outward and land with both feet wider than shoulder-width apart while swinging your arms outward and up until your hands meet over your head. Reverse these actions as you jump back to the starting position.

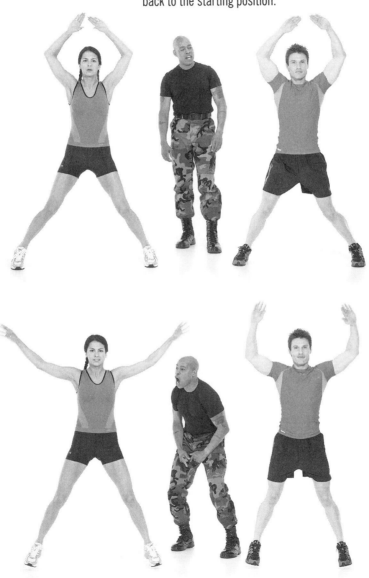

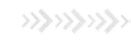

NECK STRETCH

Standing with your feet shoulder-width apart, lean your head to the left, stretching the right side. Hold for a count of 10, switch, and repeat.

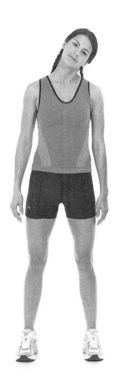
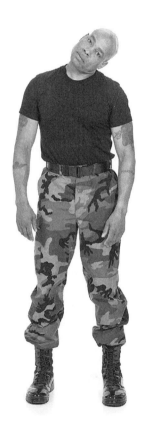
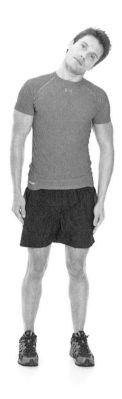

TRICEPS STRETCH

Stand with your feet shoulder-width apart. Bend the left elbow and place your left hand between your shoulder blades. Gently pull the left elbow with the right hand. Hold for a count of 10. Switch arms and repeat.

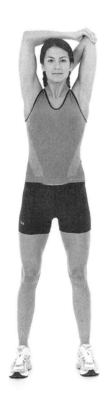
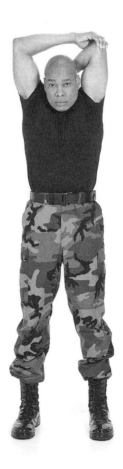
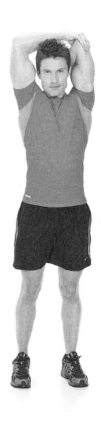

SHOULDER STRETCH

Stand with your feet shoulder-width apart. Bring your left arm across your chest and give it a gentle pull with the right hand. Hold for a count of 10. Switch arms and repeat.

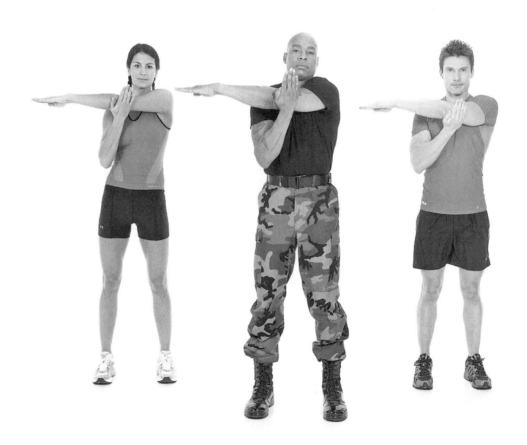

CHEST STRETCH

Stand with your feet shoulder-width apart. Clasp hands together behind the lower back with palms facing up. Pull arms toward the sky and hold for a count of 10.

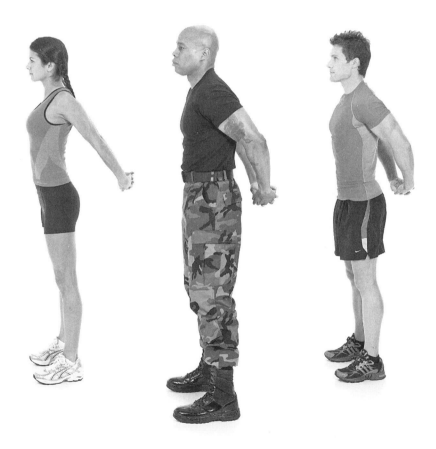

UPPER BACK STRETCH

Stand with your feet shoulder-width apart. Extend your arms in front of you at shoulder height with hands clasped and palms facing away from you. Push your arms forward, rounding your upper back while bending your knees slightly. Hold for a count of 10.

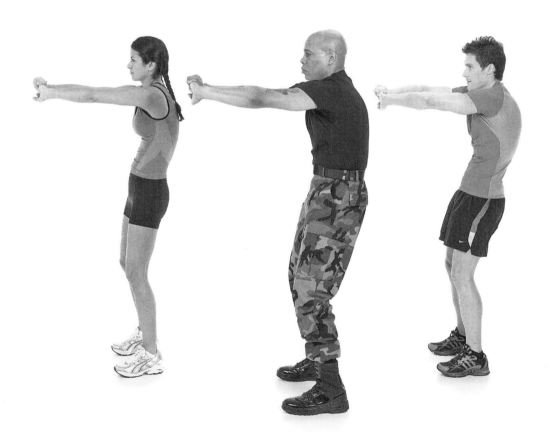

HAMSTRING STRETCH

Lie on your back. Bring your left knee toward your chest, grasping the left leg below the knee. The right knee should be slightly bent, and the right foot remains on the floor. Hold for a count of 10. Switch legs and repeat.

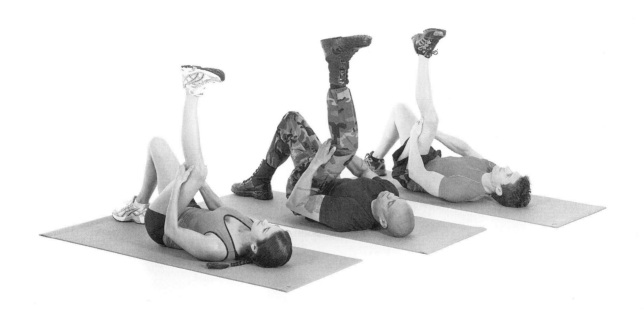

CALF STRETCH

Stand with your feet shoulder-width apart. Place your right foot in front of you, keeping both feet pointing forward and both heels on the floor. Bend the right knee slightly as you feel the stretch in the left calf. Hold for a count of 10. Switch legs and repeat.

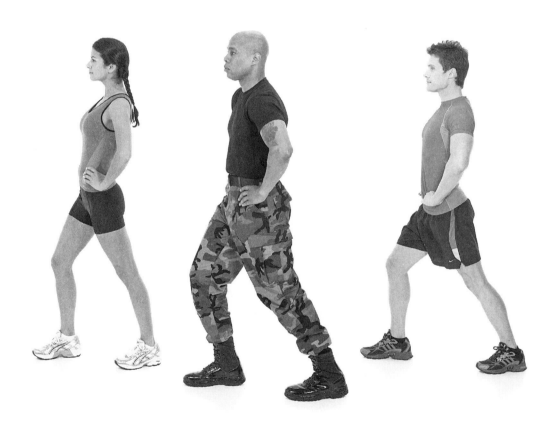

>>>>>> **GROIN STRETCH** Sitting with both knees bent and bottoms of the feet together, grasp the feet and push your knees with your elbows toward the floor. Hold for a count of 10. >>>>>>

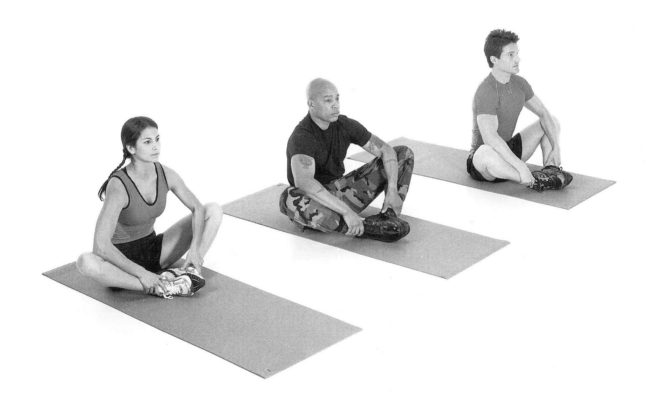

QUAD STRETCH

Lie on the floor on your right side. Grab the left ankle with the left hand and pull the left knee straight back. Hold for a count of 10. Switch legs and repeat.

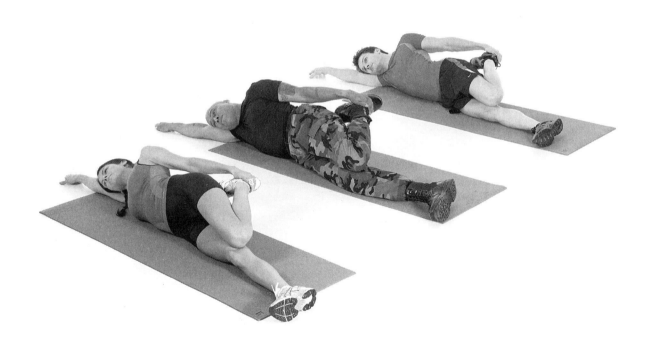

LOW BACK STRETCH

Lie on your back. Bring the left knee toward your chest, with your right leg remaining on the floor. Hold for a count of 10. Switch legs and repeat.

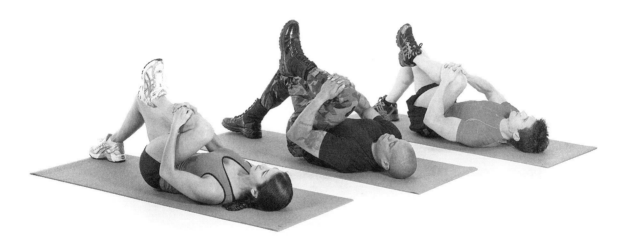

JOG ON THE SPOT (1ST GEAR)

SIDE STRADDLE HOP

Start with the feet together and hands at your side. Then jump and land with both feet wider than shoulder-width apart and bring your hands together over your head. Then jump back to the starting position.

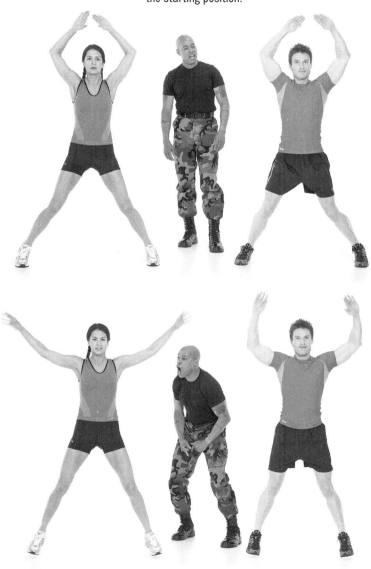

HALF JACKS

This starts in the same position as the side straddle hop. Spread your feet apart, but instead of your hands going above your head, your hands and arms will come only halfway up until they are about shoulder height, with palms facing the floor.

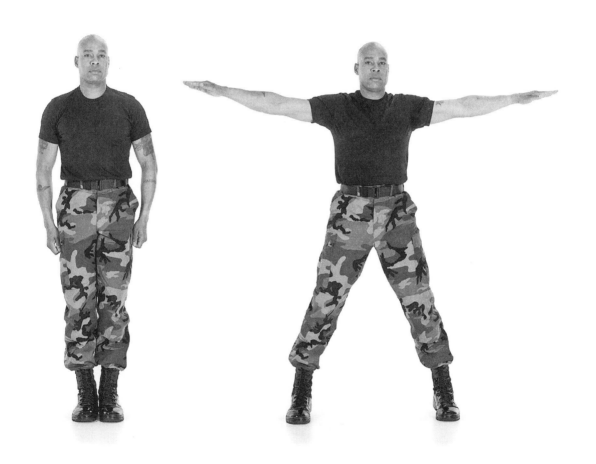

SCISSOR JACKS

Similar to cross-country skiing but without the ski poles and skis.

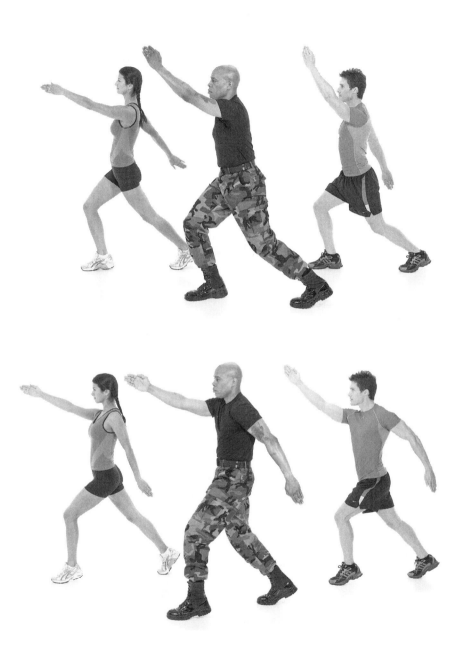

JOG ON THE SPOT (2ND GEAR)

PUSH-UPS WITH CLAP (10 REPS)

This will be done as a normal push-up with an added clap of hands as you push up off the floor.

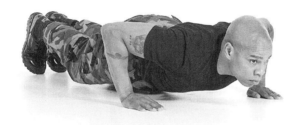

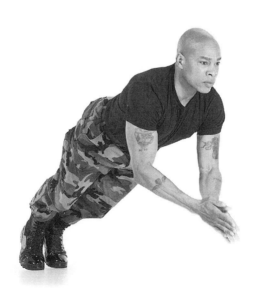

DIAMOND PUSH-UPS
(10 REPS)

Lie on your stomach. Place your hands under your chest with your index fingers of each hand and both thumbs touching, forming the shape of a diamond. All other fingers are extended. You will perform the exercise just as you would a normal push-up. When performing the push-up, raise your right foot off the ground for the first 10 reps, then lower your right foot and raise your left foot for the next 10 reps.

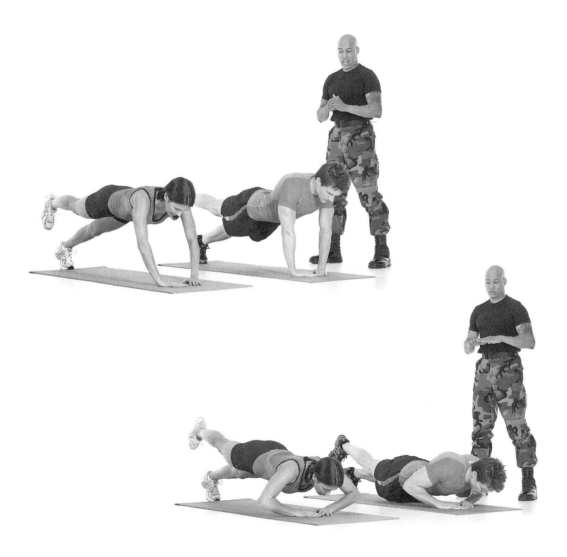

Now we are throwing in something different that will really move and tone those muscles.

Girls sometimes ask me how to deal with the roll of fat that often shows along their back when they wear a bra under a tight T-shirt. It's unsightly and it makes them feel bad about themselves.

No healthy person needs to have fat on their backs. It's put there by diet, lack of exercise, and lifestyle habits. And it can be taken away by making changes in those areas.

It's the same with men. Males tend to deposit excess fat on their gut and chest, and you can't get rid of that without taking care of all the core muscles and toning right up the core.

You can't spot-reduce the problem areas on the torso. Diet and cardiovascular work is what it needs. Take the right dietary steps, and if you work all the core muscles you're going to get the whole package.

So here are some more push-ups that will start the process, and all these variations of push-ups are money in the bank for you.

Just remember to really watch very closely where in the photos I put my hands, because correct hand placement will mean you're doing the job.

If you want to do some extra work in the gym on these problem areas, you can use light repetitions of lateral muscle pulldowns to tone the upper body, because all those muscles connect. To turn that fat into muscle, you should move onto working on high-repetition cable rolls, dumbbell rolls, and the rowing machine, all of which will build the muscle further down the line.

WIDE PUSH-UPS
(10 REPS)

Lie on your stomach. Place your hands slightly wider than shoulder-width apart with your fingers extended and each thumb joined along the hand. When performing the push-up, come to the top of the movement with your arms extended and lift your left arm and rotate your upper body to the left as far as you can go. Then place both hands back on the deck, go back down to 2 inches above the deck, and back up and lift your right arm and rotate to the right as far as you can go. That's one.

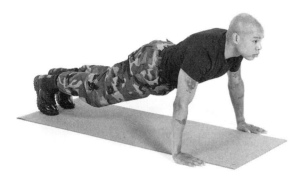

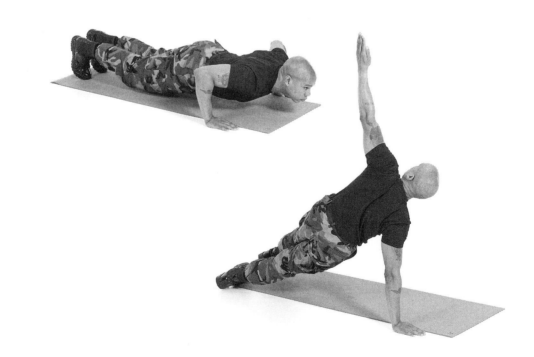

People ask me sometimes what I think of plastic surgery. I'm not a doctor, but I know everybody's doing it. I work in Los Angeles and I see it all around me.

Plastic surgery might solve some problems, but when it comes to diet and fitness, I'm a strong believer in giving yourself a fair shot and trying to do it the right way first. Why sell yourself short, taking the path of least resistance and the easy way out?

A quick fix doesn't make you fit. I've known women who have liposuction, and a year down the line the fat has all come back because they hadn't changed anything about their lives or habits.

And all operations can be dangerous.

So I say, give yourself a fair shot, try to work with your body in a natural way, and when you see good results you'll appreciate them and you'll be proud of your accomplishment. And that will build your self-esteem too.

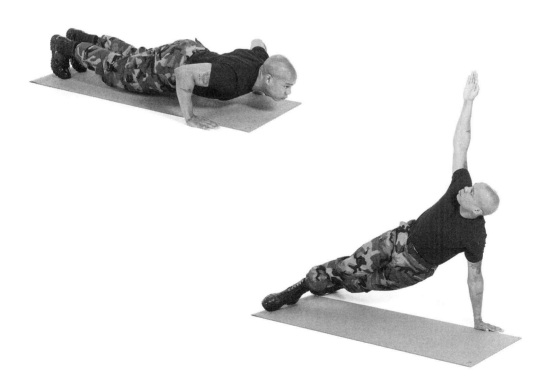

JOG ON THE SPOT (2ND GEAR) »»»»»»»»»»»»»»»»»»»»»»»»»»»»»

ARM ROTATIONS TO SIDE LATERAL FORWARD

Stand with your feet shoulder-width apart. Raise your arms until they are shoulder height, straight out to your sides, with palms facing downward. Rotate in small circles forward. Bend knees slightly and stand on the balls of your feet for the duration of the exercise. Don't forget to pull your belly button in.

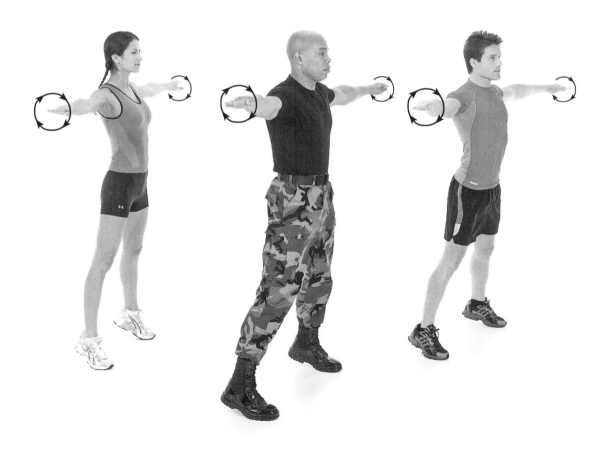

ARM ROTATIONS, FRONT

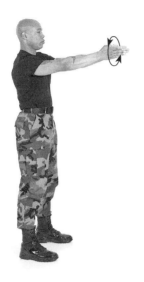

Here your arms and hands are in front of your body at shoulder height and shoulder width, with the palms of your hands facing each other. Rotate your arms outward, making small circles. Bend your knees slightly and stand on the balls of your feet for the duration of the exercise. Don't forget to pull your belly button in.

ARM ROTATIONS, OVERHEAD

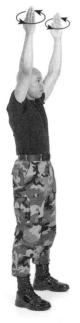

Here your arms and hands will remain straight above your head with palms facing each other. You will rotate outward, making small circles for the complete minute. Bend your knees slightly and stand on the balls of your feet for the duration of the exercise. Don't forget to pull your belly button in.

JOG ON THE SPOT (2ND GEAR) »»»»»»»»»»»»»»»»»»»»»»»»»»

4-COUNT PUSH-UPS: 2 DOWN, 2 UP

The push-ups here will be performed with hands shoulder-width apart and started in the up position. You will go down for two counts at two different levels with the chest being about 2 inches off the deck on the second count. You will then go back up to the starting position in two counts, and this completes one repetition of the exercise. You will continue to perform the exercise in this fashion for the whole minute.

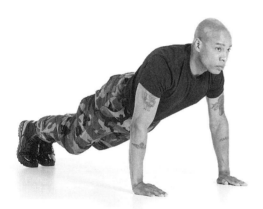
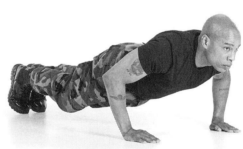
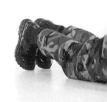

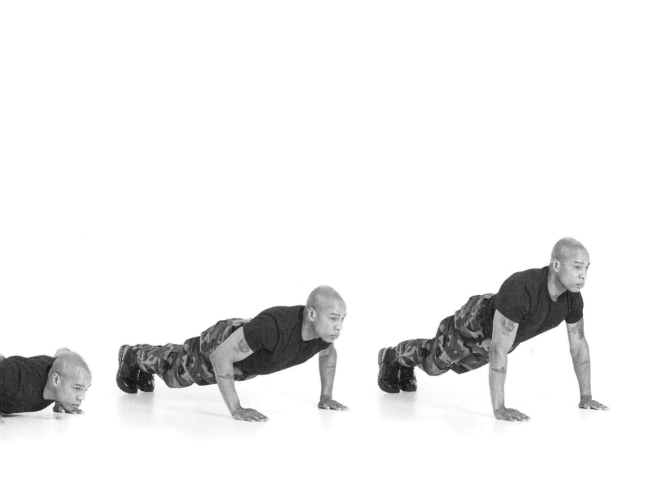

DIAMOND PUSH-UPS: 2 DOWN, 2 UP

Lie on your stomach. Place your hands under your chest with your index fingers of each hand and both thumbs touching, forming the shape of a diamond. All other fingers are extended. You will perform the exercise just as you would a normal push-up with the exception of going down in two counts and coming up in two.

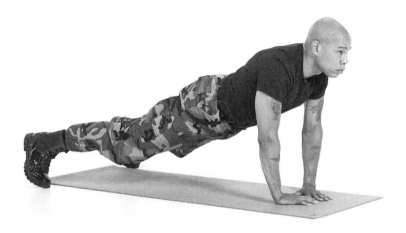

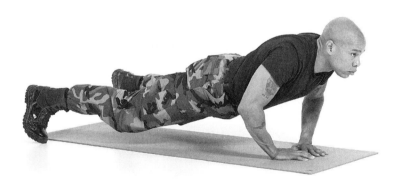

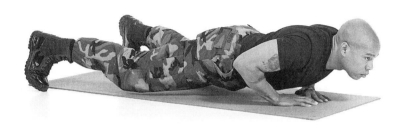

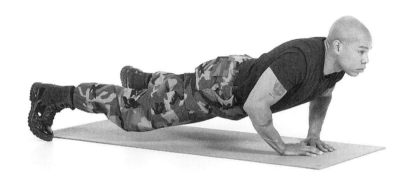

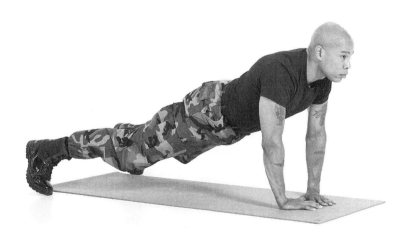

WIDE PUSH-UPS: 2 DOWN, 2 UP

Lie on your stomach. Place your hands slightly wider than shoulder-width apart with your fingers extended and each thumb joined along the hand. You will go down in two counts, with your chest about 2 inches off the deck on the second count. You will push up in two separate counts, with the second count bringing you back to the original starting position.

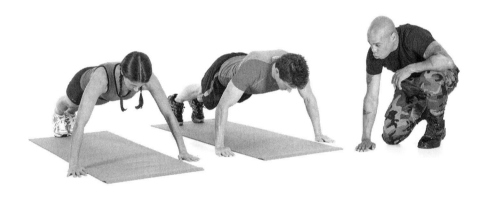

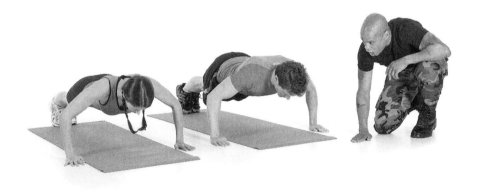

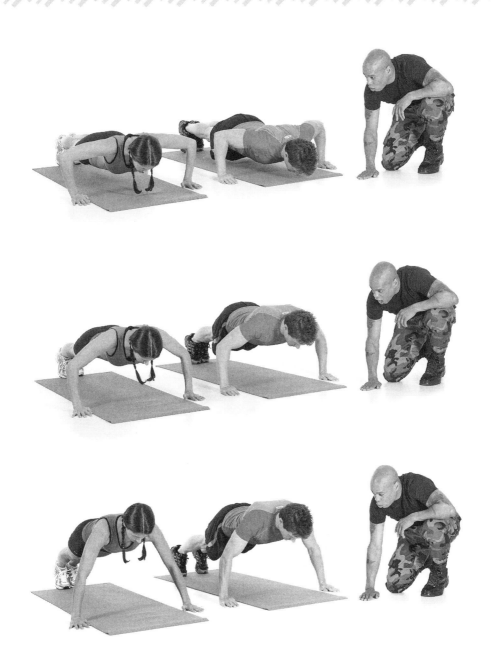

JOG ON THE SPOT (2ND GEAR) >>>>>>>>>>>>>>>>>>>>>>>>>>>>>>>>>>>>>>

4-COUNT BEAT BOOTS: 3 DOWN, 1 UP

Stand with your feet shoulder-width apart. Extend your arms in front of the body at shoulder height. Squat down for three counts by bending the knees a little more at each level and keeping your belly button pulled in and your weight on your heels. On the third count, lower your hands to your sides and reach around and tap your ankles. Once ankles are tapped, you will stand completely up in one count while raising your arms so that they are again extended in front of you at shoulder height, completing one repetition of the exercise.

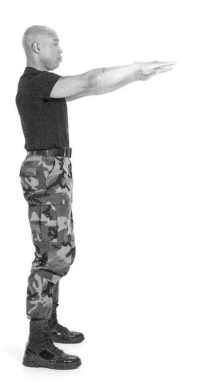
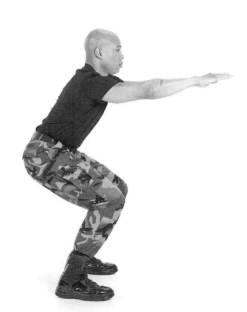

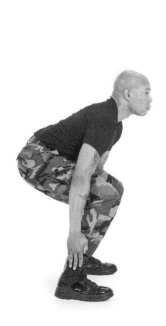

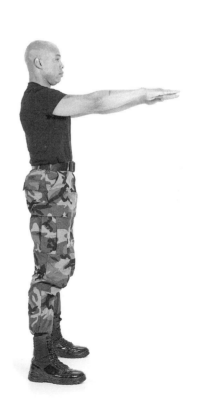

LEFT LEG CROSS LUNGE

Stand with your feet shoulder-width apart. Move your left leg across your right leg, landing your heel on the floor. Continue to lunge, working the left leg for the complete minute.

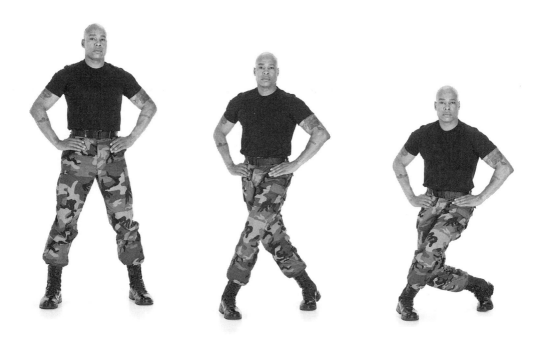

When people ask me what to do about problem areas on the thighs, I tell them to do lunges. This exercise will tone your thigh muscles, strengthen your balance, and you will feel and see the difference if you stay at it, take the right dietary steps, and keep working it off.

I know these exercises are hard, but if you've made it to Stage Three, you'll know that, although you might not see much happening, your body is changing—for the better. If you want to keep those changes coming, keep doing it. Follow the program. Trust me, you'll see a difference sooner than you think.

Lunges will help shape up your hips and butt too—as long as you stay in the fight and keep it going.

RIGHT LEG CROSS LUNGE

Stand with your feet shoulder-width apart. Move your right leg across your left leg, landing your heel on the floor. Continue to lunge, working the right leg for the complete minute.

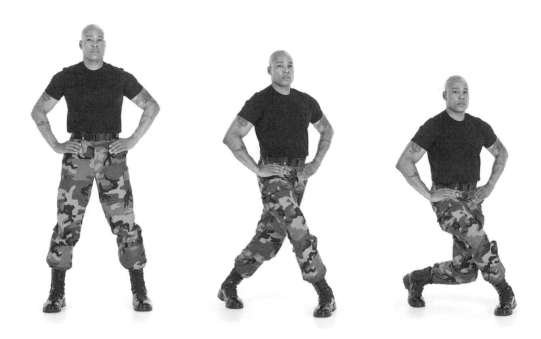

If the hip area is a problem for you, it can help to do some extra work on steps. Everybody has access to stairs somewhere and taking steps up and down works the glutes and quads—those muscles around your butt and thighs—extremely well.

So take advantage and schedule another little session just on stepping. If you're doing the full workout four times a week as well, you'll be fit enough to take on a little extra.

This isn't about a one-off or a weekend. This is a change of your whole lifestyle. That's what will solve these problem areas.

SINGLE CALF RAISE: LEFT CALF

This will be performed with the left foot on the floor first and the right foot slightly lifted off the deck and placed behind the left, slightly touching outside of the left ankle. Lift up on the toes with a two count and back down with a two count.

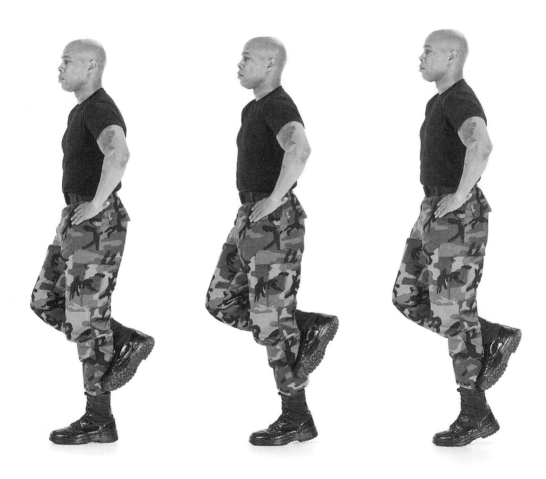

SINGLE CALF RAISE: RIGHT CALF

This will be performed with the right foot on the floor and the left foot slightly lifted off the floor and wrapped behind the right leg, slightly touching outside of the right ankle. Lift up on the toes with a two count and back down with a two count.

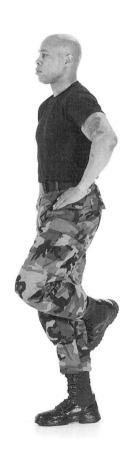 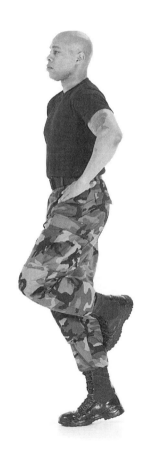 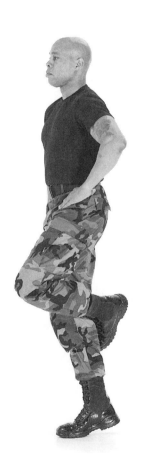

JOG ON THE SPOT (3RD GEAR) »»»»»»»»»»»»»»

BODY TWISTS WITH LEGS STRAIGHT

Lie on your back with your arms extended straight out from your shoulders. Legs will be straight up at a 90-degree angle, with the bottom of your feet facing straight up to the sky. Starting to the left, rotate both feet to the left, then back to center, then to the right, in a controlled motion. Continue rotating for the full 1 minute.

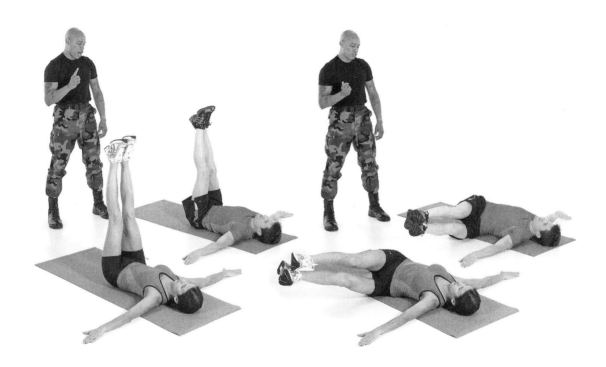

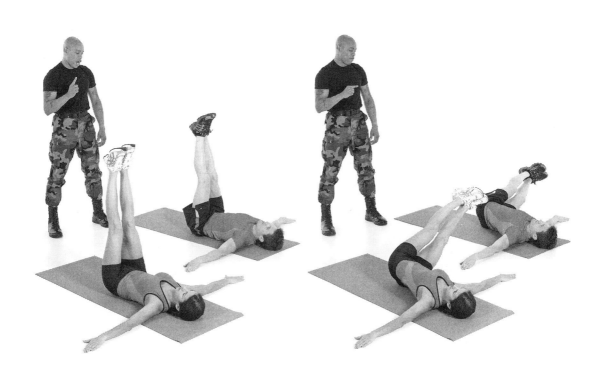

4-COUNT LEG LIFTS

Lie on your back with your legs extended, raising your feet 6 inches off the floor, with your toes pointing away from you. You may place your hands under your butt for support. Raise your feet up for a count of two, ending with your feet pointing toward the sky and legs at a 90-degree angle, then lower your legs down in two counts until your feet are 6 inches off the floor again.

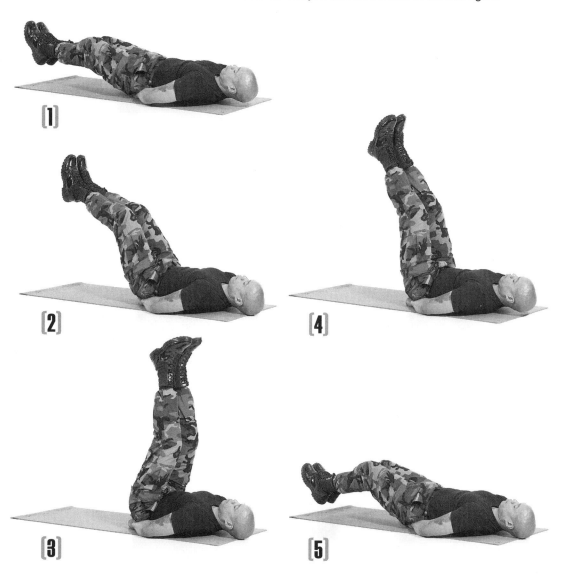

[1]

[2]

[3]

[4]

[5]

FLUTTER KICKS

Lie on your back with your legs extended, raising your feet 6 inches off the floor, with your toes pointing away from you. You may place your hands under your butt for support. Start with your left leg and then alternate with the right as if you were swimming. Your feet should never touch the floor.

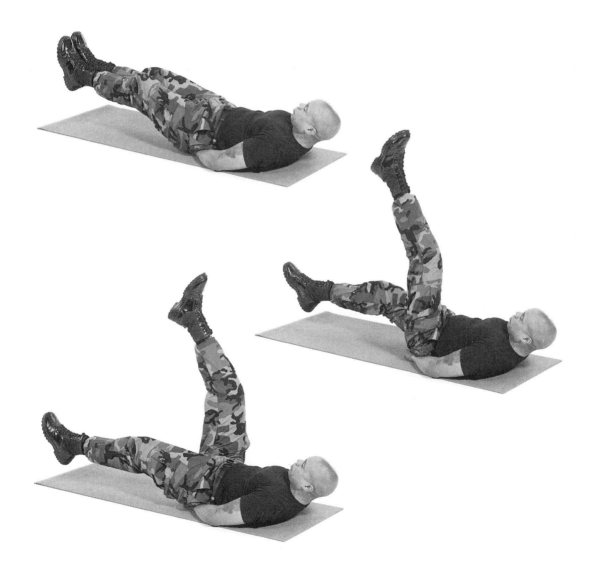

4-COUNT HELLO SUNSHINES

Lie on your back with your legs extended, raising your feet 6 inches off the floor, with your toes pointing away from you. On four counts you will start to separate your feet, spreading your legs apart and keeping your feet 6 inches off the floor throughout the whole exercise. After the fourth count, bring your feet back together in one motion.

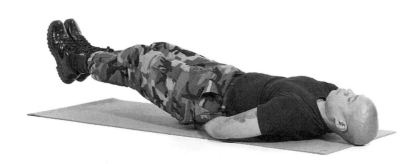

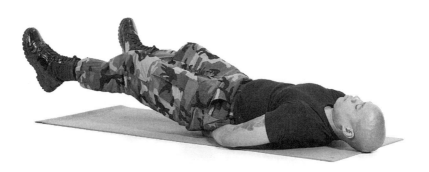

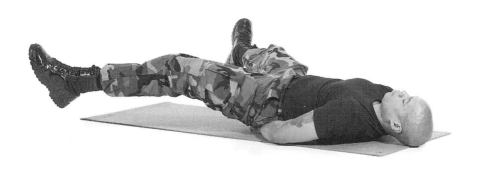

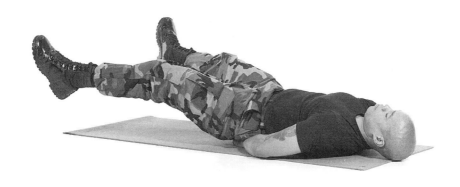

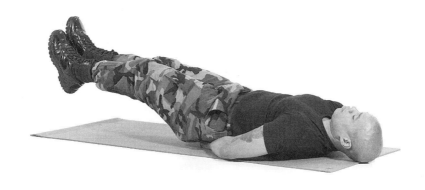

JOG ON THE SPOT (3RD GEAR) ≫≫≫≫≫≫≫≫≫≫≫≫≫≫≫≫≫≫

HARD-CORE HARVEY BUILDERS
WITH ARM ROTATIONS

Stand straight with your feet together and your arms extended to your sides at shoulder height. Make big circles forward for 30 rotations. Now make 30 rotations backward. Immediately after the arm rotations, squat all the way down, touching the floor with your hands on the outside of your feet. Kick both feet out behind you, placing you in a push-up position. You will now perform four regular push-ups, then kick your feet back into the squat position and stand up. After the arm rotations, the first count is the squat, second count is the feet kicking back, third count is the down feet coming back in, placing you in squat position with your hands on the outside of each foot, and the fourth position will be you standing up into the starting point for one repetition. Keep performing this sequence for the complete minute.

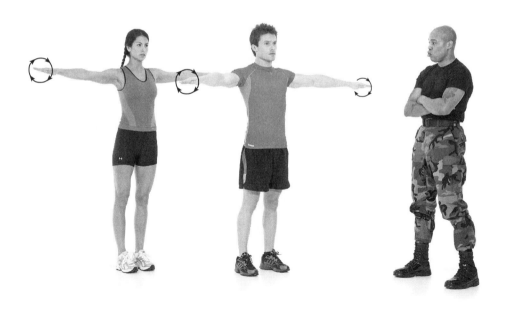

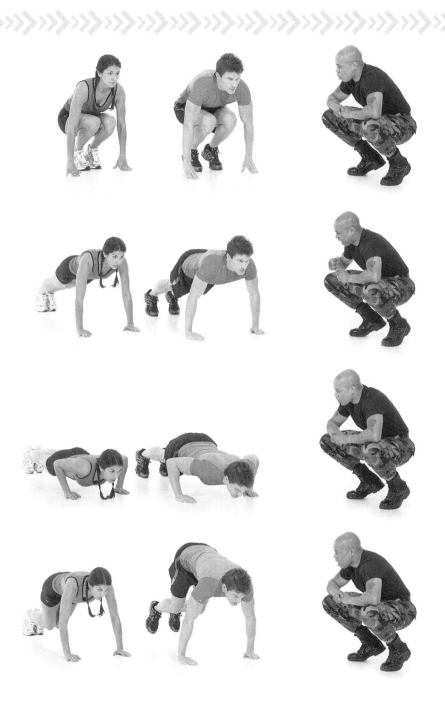

JOG ON THE SPOT (3RD GEAR) >>>>>>>>>>>>>>>>>>>>>>>>>>>>>>>>>

JOG ON THE SPOT (2ND GEAR) (3 MINUTES)

JOG ON THE SPOT (1ST GEAR) (1 MINUTE)

MARCH ON THE SPOT (1 MINUTE)

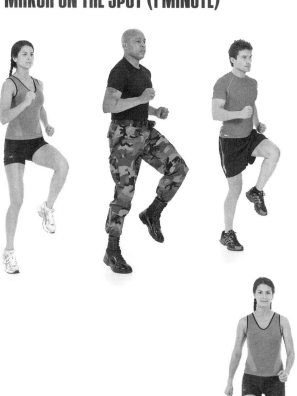

NECK STRETCH

Standing with feet shoulder-width apart, lean your head to the left, stretching the right side. Hold for a count of 20, switch, and repeat.

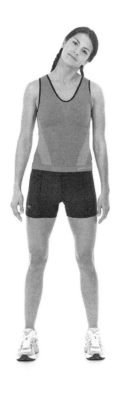
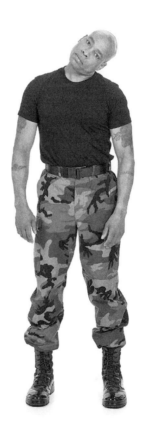
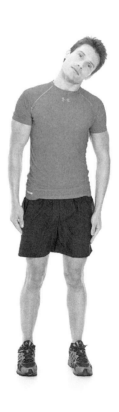

TRICEPS STRETCH

Stand with your feet shoulder-width apart. Bend the left elbow and place your left hand between your shoulder blades. Gently pull the left elbow with the right hand. Hold for a count of 20. Switch arms and repeat.

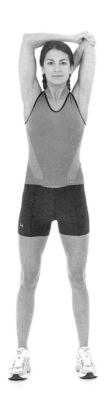
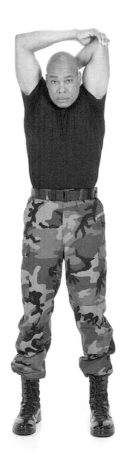
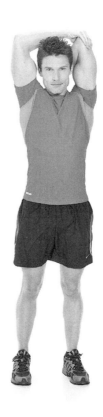

>>>>>> **SHOULDER STRETCH** Stand with your feet shoulder-width apart. Bring your left arm across your chest and give a gentle pull with the right hand. Hold for a count of 20. Switch arms and repeat. >>>>>

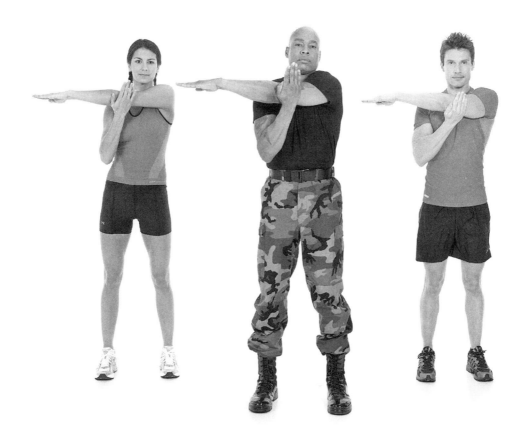

CHEST STRETCH

Stand with your feet shoulder-width apart. Clasp your hands together behind the lower back, with palms facing up. Pull your arms toward the sky and hold for a count of 20.

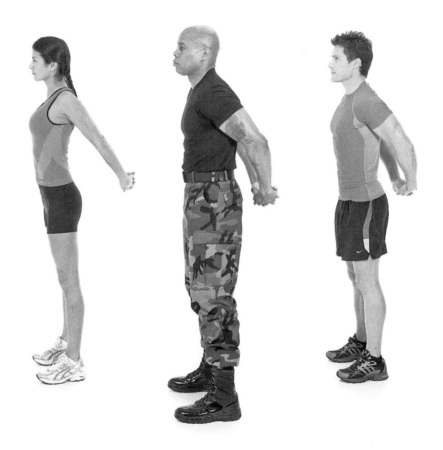

UPPER BACK STRETCH

Stand with your feet shoulder-width apart. Extend your arms in front of you at shoulder height with your hands clasped and palms facing away from you. Push your arms forward, rounding the upper back while bending your knees slightly. Hold for a count of 20.

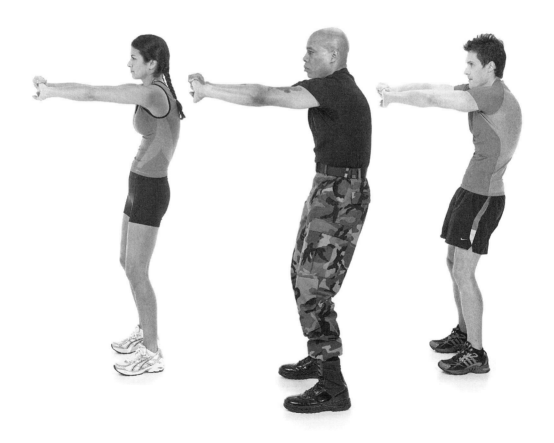

HAMSTRING STRETCH

Lie on your back. Bring your left knee toward your chest, grasping the left leg below the knee. The right knee should be slightly bent and the right foot remains on the floor. Hold for a count of 20. Switch legs and repeat.

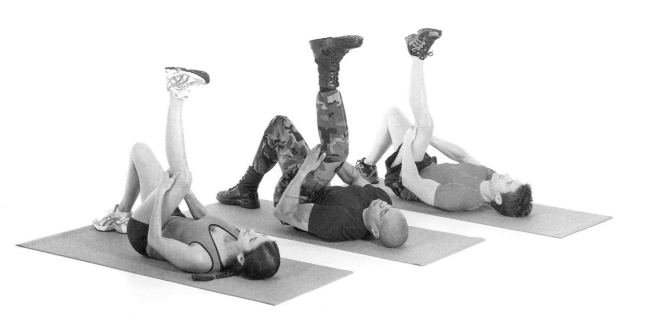

CALF STRETCH

Stand with your feet shoulder-width apart. Place your right foot in front of you, keeping both feet pointing forward and both heels on the floor. Bend the right knee slightly as you feel the stretch in the left calf. Hold for a count of 20. Switch legs and repeat.

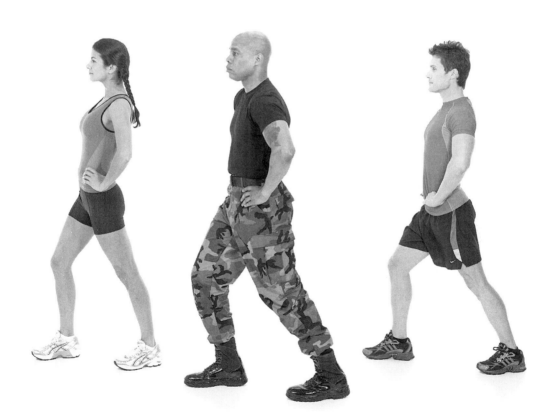

GROIN STRETCH

Sitting with both knees bent and bottoms of the feet together, grasp the feet and push your knees, with your elbows toward the floor. Hold for a count of 20.

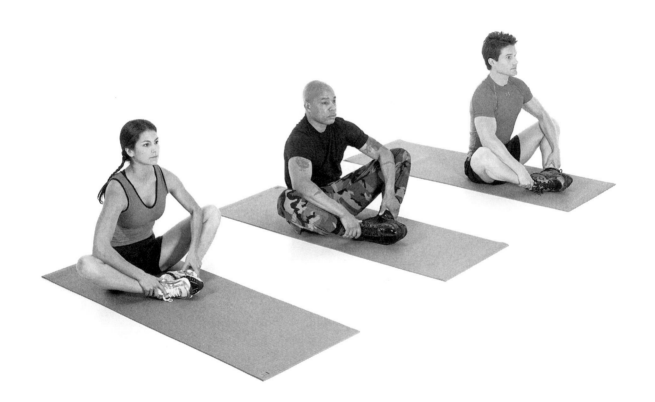

QUAD STRETCH

Lie on the floor on your right side. Grab the left ankle with the left hand and pull the left knee straight back. Hold for a count of 20. Switch legs and repeat.

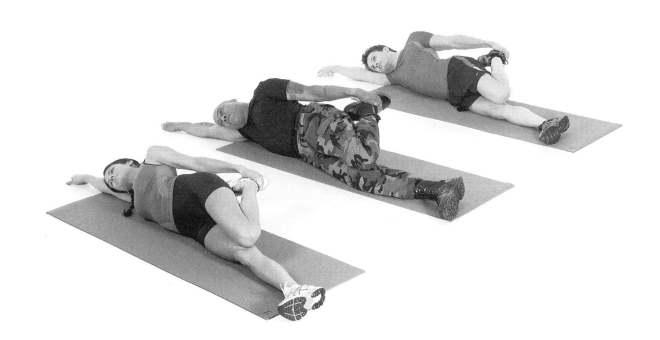

LOW BACK STRETCH

Lie on your back. Bring your left knee toward your chest, with your right leg remaining on the floor. Hold for a count of 20. Switch legs and repeat.

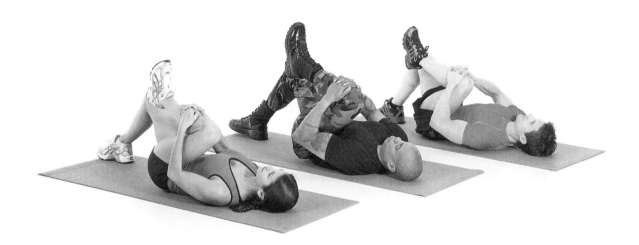

And if you have come this far, you have reached the

Harvey Walden supersonic

fitness suite, and you've shown that you've got

discipline, drive, and energy and you can stick to it. You've gone

through your personal wall and you've gotten over your issues.

You've climbed that hill

and you know your own

strength. You've accomplished something.

WELCOME
ABOARD.

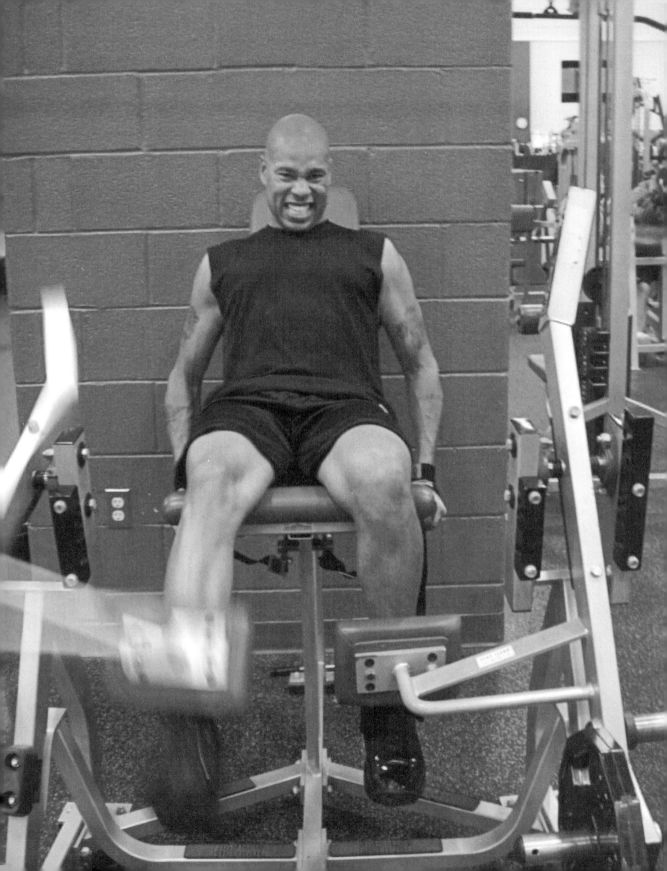

7

BONUS GYM SECTION

For you gym rats looking for exercises to target certain muscles, these are some of my favorites.

HANGING KNEE LIFTS

An overhead pull-up bar is required for this exercise. Hanging on the bar with a wide grip, lift your legs and knees toward your chest using a slow, controlled raise and try to limit upper-body movement. Hold the raised position, and lower your legs in a controlled movement and repeat.

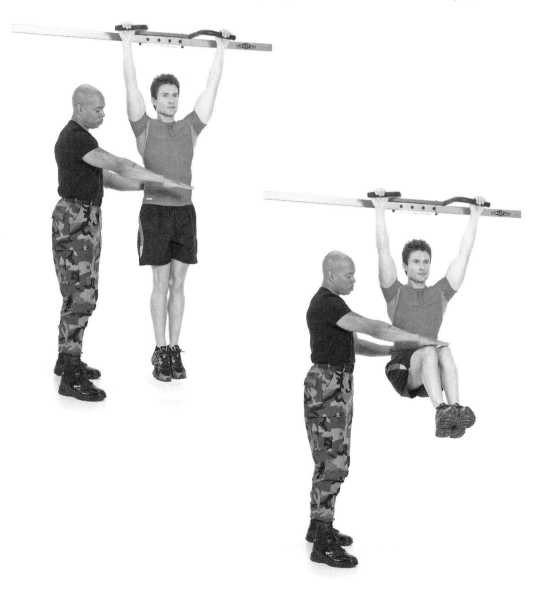

CRUNCHES ON EXERCISE BALL

Sit on top of an exercise ball with your feet placed on the floor. Roll on the ball until your lower back is centered on top of the ball. Place your hands behind your ears and crunch your upper body forward. Then lower your back to the starting position and repeat.

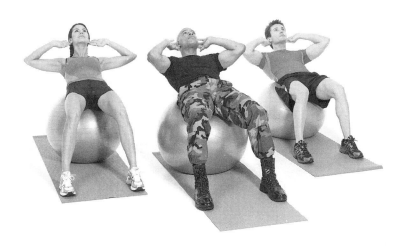

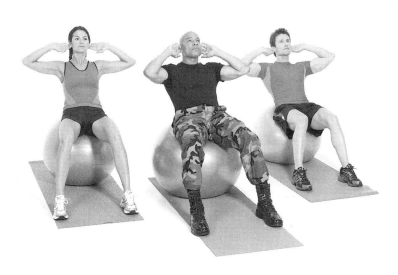

OBLIQUE CRUNCHES ON EXERCISE BALL

Sit on top of an exercise ball with your feet placed on the floor. Roll on the ball until your lower back is centered on top of the ball. Place your hands behind your ears and crunch your upper body forward, first turning to the right side and then repeating the move but turning toward the left side.

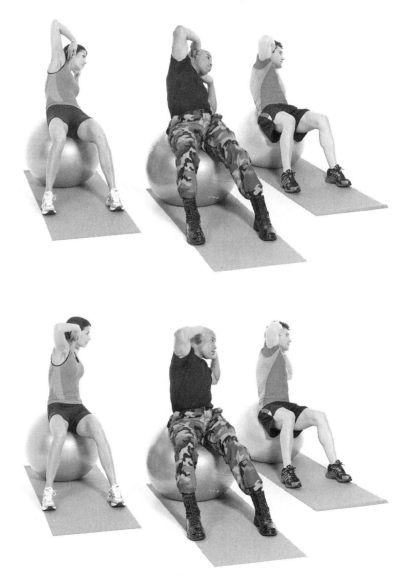

EZ CURLS

Select the correct weights for your strength and stand (knees slightly bent) holding the EZ curl bar with both hands shoulder-width apart with an underhand grip.

With the bar hanging at arm's length (almost touching the tops of your legs), curl the bar up until your forearms touch your biceps. Keep your elbows close to your sides at all times.

Use a slow, controlled curl and keep your back straight and upright at all times.

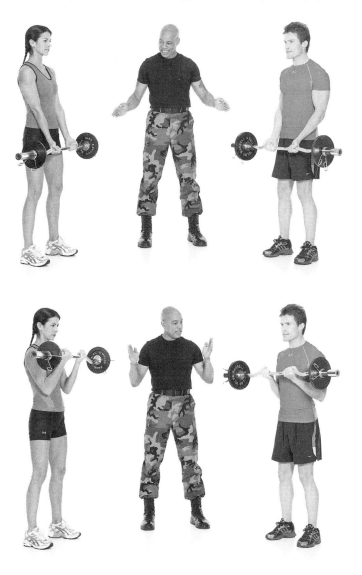

SEATED DUMBBELL CURLS

Sit on the end of a shoulder- or chest-press bench and take a dumbbell with your desired weight in each hand.

Hold the dumbbells at your side extended to arm's length with your palms turned toward your body.

One at a time, curl the weights forward and up, twisting your palms forward as you lift so that the thumbs turn to the outside and the palms are facing up. Remember to use a slow, controlled curl.

Curl the dumbbells up until your forearms touch your biceps.

Lower the dumbbells down through the same movement, resisting the weight all the way down until your arms are fully extended, and repeat.

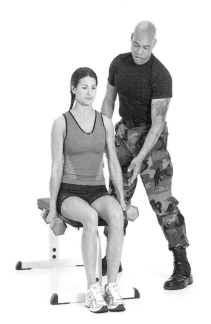

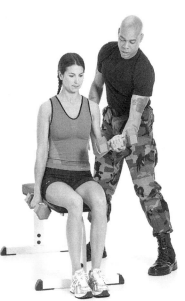

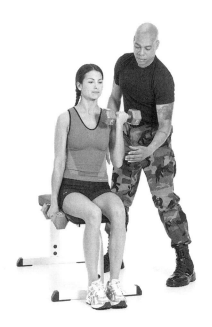

PREACHER CURLS

To perform this exercise you will require a weight bench with a preacher curl attachment. (Some gyms may have a preacher curl machine.)

With your desired weights added, hold the barbell with your palms facing up.

Sit on the bench and place your elbows on the preacher curl pad.

Extend arms fully until the fronts of your forearms are touching the curl pad.

Keeping your elbows on the pad, curl the barbell toward your body, maintaining a slow, controlled curl until your forearms touch your biceps.

Lower the barbell down through the same movement, resisting the weight all the way down until your arms are fully extended, and repeat.

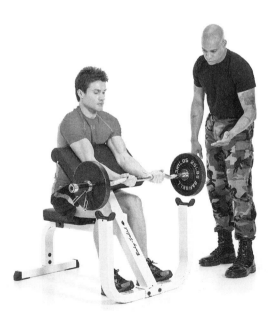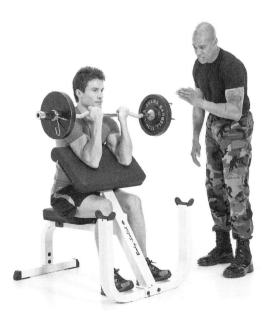

DUMBBELL HAMMER CURLS

Select the desired weight for your dumbbells and stand straight with your feet shoulder-width apart. Your arms should be fully extended by your sides and your palms facing toward your body.

Using one arm at a time, raise until your forearm is parallel with the floor, pause, and lower the dumbbell down through the same movement, resisting the weight all the way down, until your arm is fully extended. Repeat with the opposite arm.

Remember to keep your back straight.

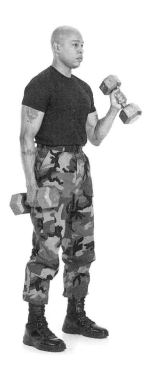
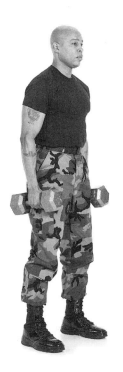
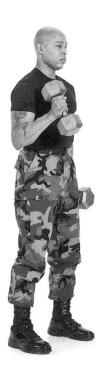

ONE-ARM DUMBBELL EXTENSIONS

This one-arm dumbbell extension can be performed either standing or seated, whichever you find more comfortable. Take a dumbbell, select your desired weights, and hold in either your right or left arm. Raise your arm up until it is fully extended with your palm facing forward.

Once the arm is fully extended, slowly bend the elbow and lower the dumbbell down behind your neck, keeping a controlled movement.

Raise the dumbbell back through the same movement, resisting the weight to the starting position, and repeat. Once you have performed your desired number of reps, perform the same exercise with the opposite arm.

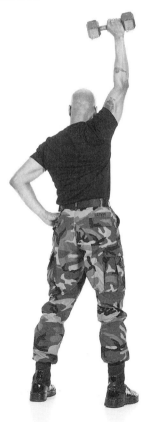
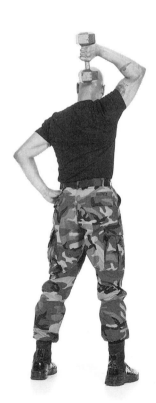

ARMS

ONE-ARM CABLE PUSH-DOWNS

For this exercise you will require a standing cable machine.

Standing in front of the machine, grasp the cable handle using an underhand grip.

Start the movement with the handle close to your chin. Keeping a slow, controlled movement, push the weight down to your waist until your arm is fully extended, keeping your elbow at your side.

Raise the cable back through the same movement, resisting the weight to the starting position and repeat. Once you have performed your desired number of reps, perform the same exercise with the opposite arm.

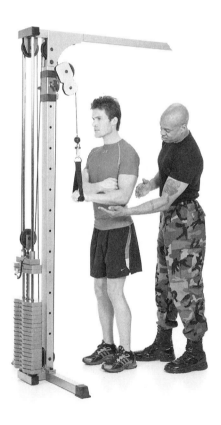 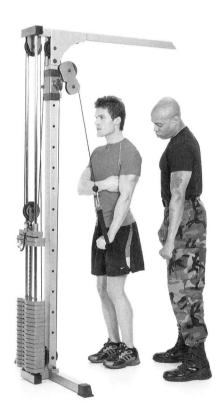

TWO-HAND TRICEPS PUSH-DOWNS

For this exercise you will require a standing cable machine with a straight bar to grip.

Standing in front of the machine, grasp the straight bar with both hands palms down, slightly less than shoulder-width apart.

Start the movement with the bar close to your chin. Keeping a slow, controlled movement, push the bar down to your waist until your arms are fully extended, keeping your elbows at your sides.

Raise the bar back through the same movement, resisting the weight to the starting position, and repeat.

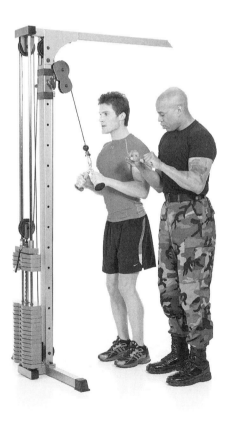 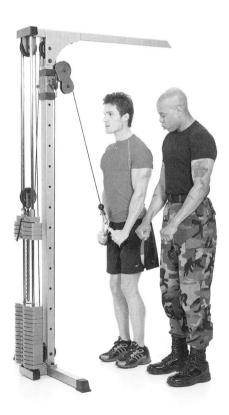

LEG PRESS

For this exercise you will require a leg press machine.

Select your desired weights and sit on the leg press machine with your back straight against the back pad.

Place your feet on the press, keeping your knees slightly bent.

Under control, push and extend your legs before your knees lock, pause, and reverse the movement back, resisting the weight until you are back to that start position and then repeat.

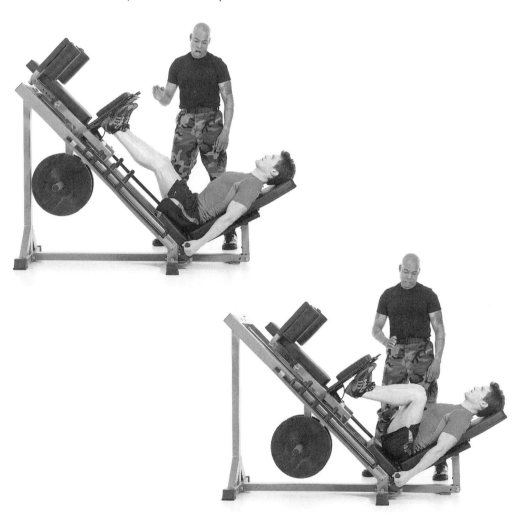

HACK SQUAT

For this exercise you will require a hack squat machine.

Select your desired weights and sit on the hack squat machine with your back straight against the back pad.

Place your feet just over shoulder-width apart and begin this exercise by squatting, controlling the weight until your knees reach a 90-degree angle and your thighs become parallel to the push deck.

Hold this position, then return to the start position in a controlled movement and repeat.

As this movement can be quite intense and uses heavy weights, it is always advisable to have an instructor or friend acting as a spotter.

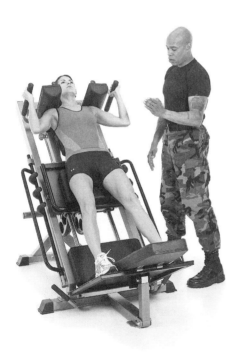
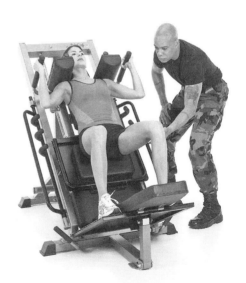

LEGS/GLUTES

LEG CURL

For this exercise you will require a leg curl machine.

Select your desired weights and lie facedown on the leg curl machine, gripping the underneath handles.

Place the back of your ankles under the curl pad and curl your legs up, keeping your hips down against the bench.

Once you have reached the top of the curl, slowly lower the weight back in a controlled movement to the start position and repeat.

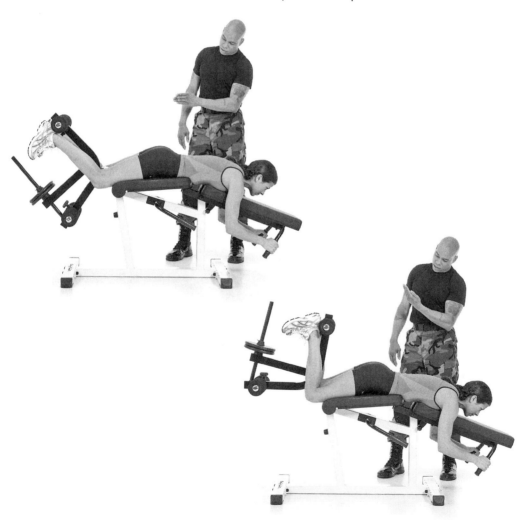

CALF RAISES

For this exercise you will require the seated or standing calf raise machine.

Select your desired weight. If using the seated machine place knees under pad, and with your toes, lift up and hold for a count of two and lower.

If using the standing machine, use the same concept as sitting, just ensure your feet are shoulder-width apart and place shoulders under pads.

Hold the position, then lower, returning to the start position and repeat.

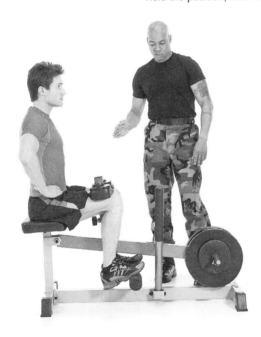

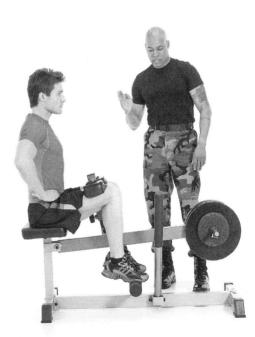

DUMBBELL LUNGES

Select your desired weights for your dumbbells and stand with both arms fully extended to your sides with your palms facing toward your body.

Standing with your feet shoulder-width apart, lunge forward with your first leg landing on your heel and then your forefoot. Ideally you want both knees to be at about 90-degree angles at the bottom of the movement.

Return to the start position and repeat exercise with the opposite leg.

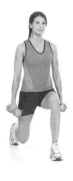
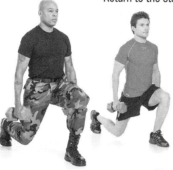

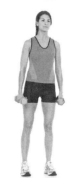
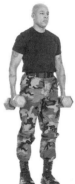
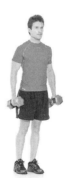

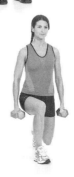
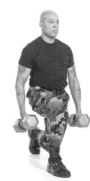
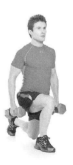

SEATED DUMBBELL PRESSES

Select your desired weights and sit on a shoulder press bench with your back straight against the back pad.

Take a dumbbell in each hand and raise the dumbbells up until the back section of your arms (triceps) are parallel to the floor. Your palms should be facing forward and the weights should now be in line with your head.

Keep your feet planted firmly on the ground and push the weights up straight over your head (do not lock your elbows), pause, and under control, reverse the movement back, resisting the weight until you are back to that start position and then repeat.

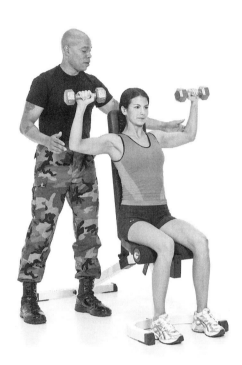

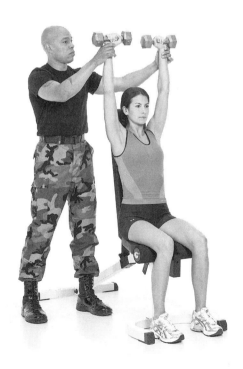

SHOULDERS

STANDING SIDE LATERAL RAISES

Select your desired weights and stand with your feet shoulder-width apart.

Hold the dumbbells in front of your waist with your elbows slightly bent and your palms facing in toward each other.

Simultaneously raise the dumbbells upward and out to your sides.

Raise your arms until they are both parallel to the floor, pause, and then, under control, reverse the movement back, resisting the weight until you are back to the start position and then repeat.

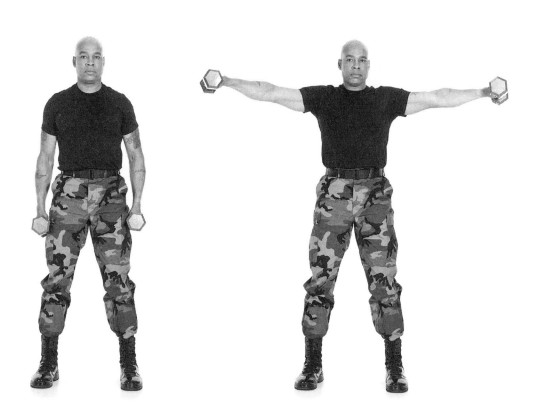

FLAT BENCH DUMBBELL PRESSES

Select your desired weights and lie back on a flat press bench.

Keep your feet planted firmly on the ground and simultaneously raise the dumbbells until the backs of your upper arms (triceps) are parallel with the floor.

Push the dumbbells up over your chest with the elbows to the sides, until your arms are fully extended (do not lock your elbows), pause, and, under control, reverse the movement back, resisting the weight until you are back to the start position and then repeat.

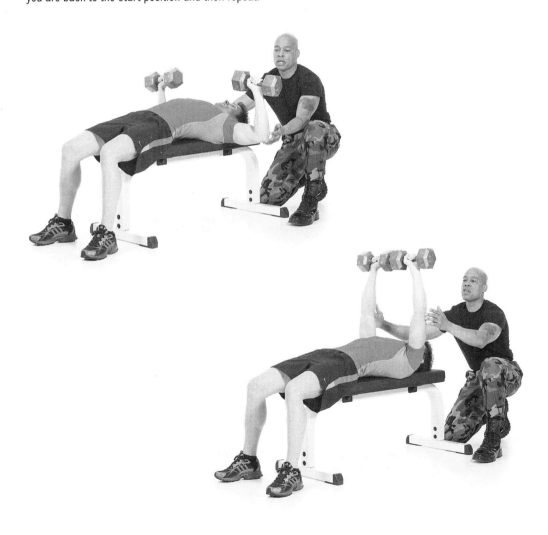

SEATED CHEST-PRESS MACHINE

For this exercise you will require a seated chest-press machine.

Select your desired weights and sit on the chest-press machine.

Adjust the seat until your chest is just above the horizontal push handles. Keep your back straight against the back pad.

If available, push the foot lever until the push handles are at a comfortable position to grip.

Grasp the handles with an overhand grip, release the foot lever, and push the weight.

Push the weight until your arms are fully extended (but not locked), pause, and, under control, reverse the movement back, resisting the weight until you are back to the start position and then repeat.

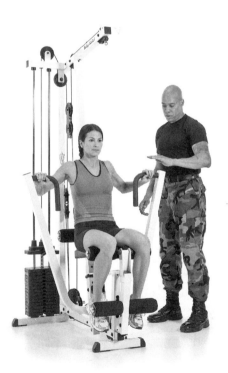
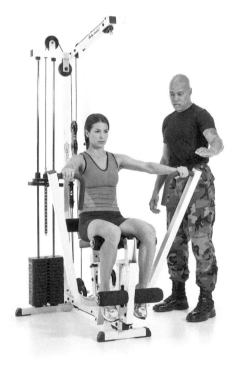

INCLINE BENCH PRESS/DUMBBELLS

Select your desired weights and sit on an incline bench with an incline just under 45 degrees.

Keep your feet planted firmly on the ground, and simultaneously raise the dumbbells until the backs of your upper arms (triceps) are parallel with the floor.

Push the dumbbells up over your chest with the elbows to the sides until your arms are fully extended (do not lock your elbows), pause, and, under control, reverse the movement back, resisting the weight until you are back to the start position and then repeat.

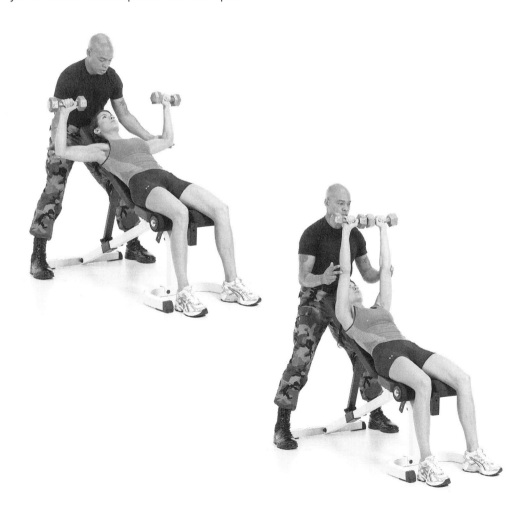

DUMBBELL FLYS

Select your desired weights and lie back on a flat press bench.

Keep your feet planted firmly on the ground and simultaneously raise the dumbbells until your arms are fully extended with the dumbbells over your chest and your palms facing toward each other.

Slowly lower your arms down and out to your sides until your chest muscles are stretched and your arms are parallel to the floor, pause, and, under control, reverse the movement back, resisting the weight until you are back to the start position and then repeat.

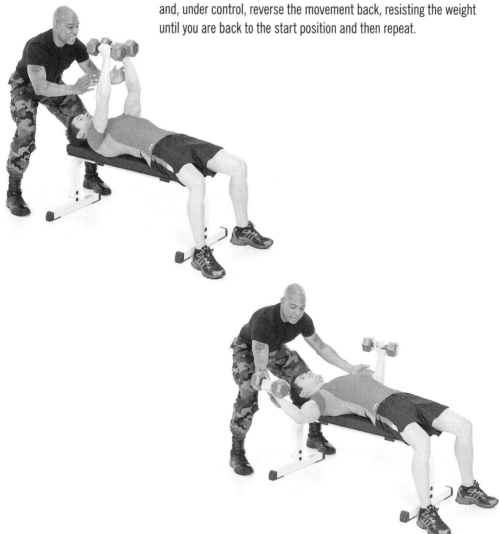

FRONT LAT PULL-DOWN

For this exercise you will require a lat pull-down machine.

Select your desired weights and sit at the lat pull-down machine with your thighs under the supports.

Grasp the straight pull bar with a wide grip with your palms facing away.

Start with your arms fully extended upward, and with your back straight, begin to pull the bar straight down until it touches your chest, pause, and, under control, reverse the movement back, resisting the weight until you are back to the start position and then repeat.

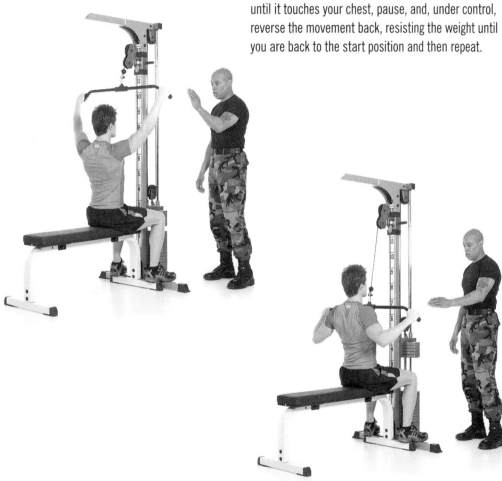

SEATED CABLE ROW

For this exercise you will require a low cable machine.

Select your desired weights and sit on the platform with your knees bent and grasp the cable attachment or handles. Your arms should be fully extended (but not locked).

Keeping your back straight, slowly pull the cable attachment/handles toward your body, until your hands almost touch your torso, pause, and, under control, reverse the movement back, resisting the weight until you are back to the start position and then repeat.

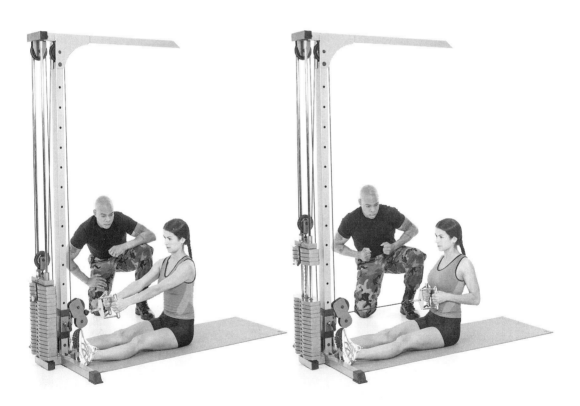

BENT-OVER DUMBBELL ROW

Select your desired weights and kneel over a flat bench with one arm holding the dumbbell, leg to one side, and your other arm supporting your weight on the bench.

Under control, pull the dumbbell up to your side/stomach and hold the position when your elbow is in line with your shoulder.

Under control, reverse the movement back, resisting the weight until you are back to the start position and then repeat.

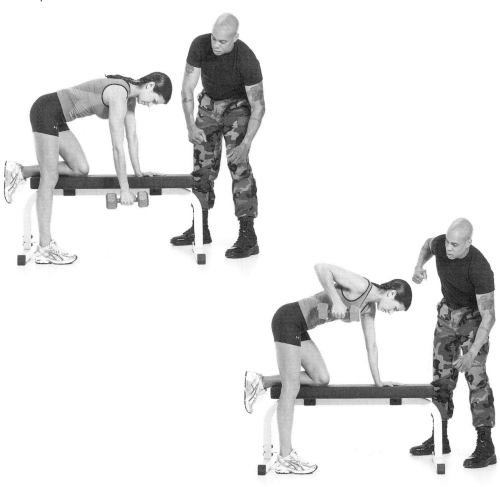

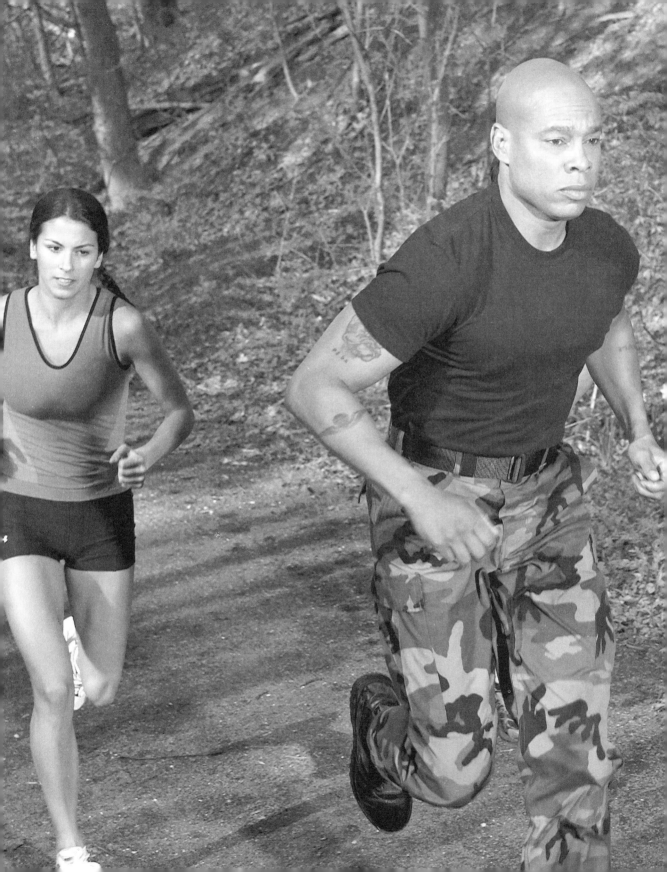

8

HARVEY'S HIDDEN MOTIVATOR

So what I'm saying to you is: Find your hidden motivator. Find the thing that works for you. The thing that pulls your hidden heartstrings. Hey, I'm a tough marine and I train warriors. I'm not playing softball. All I mean is: Everybody's got something they'll die for.

And when you know what that something is, you'll know what you really live for, too.

So lean on your secret motivator. Keep it in front of you. As I've said, I like to keep a picture of Halle Berry in my workout diary. She inspires me because she's a survivor and a great person. Looking at that picture helps me pick myself up when I'm feeling low.

We can all surround ourselves with positive motivators that work for us.

Some people keep pictures. Others prefer words close by them, to give them strength and inspiration. Maybe a letter or card from a loved one. Or maybe it's your dog that does it for you. In the marines I've seen all kinds of things that give fighting men their courage. But there is one thing I know. Everyone's got something that presses their buttons.

Whatever yours is, you will know. Whatever inspires you, or means something to you, and gives you the encouragement you need to go make some money, that's what you need to look at, that's what you need to keep by you and work with. Don't be shy. This is for you and you alone, and it don't mean nothing to no one else. It's your life and YOU are in control.

I'm not telling you what to do—the choice is yours. What I'm saying is: Dig deep, grasshopper, and find your personal power.

And when you've found what it is in your life that keeps you going along that track, stay with it. Be loyal to your inspiration, hold on to your motivators, keep them in mind, keep sight of your goal, and you'll accomplish more.

The thing that keeps me going most of all is no secret. My two kids, Tiyauna and Harvey, are my perfect motivators.

Being there for the birth of Harvey V, November 30, Moline, Illinois, about two hours outside of Chicago, was the best thing a man could ask for. It was special for me because I'd been deployed when my daughter was born and didn't see her until she was a year old, and that was kind of gut-wrenching. I guess that was the first time in my life I actually cried, and they were tears of joy.

I was always a tough cookie. But on that day, when that little baby cried his first cry, my newborn son, so small that I could measure his whole forearm with just one of my doggone fingers, I went into the bathroom so that no one would see and smiled through my own tears.

Shoot, I can't begin to describe how proud I was. I'd kept praying all along that I would have a son, and sure enough, it happened. Here he was. Harvey Walden V. The first son. That was definitely money in the bank there.

I took my kids everywhere I could when they were little. Harvey and I watched the Chicago Bulls win a championship together. It was Harvey's first game. He had his first little Chicago

Bulls T-shirt when he was still in grade school. And Tiyauna was always a daddy's girl. Everywhere I went she would tag along with me. She was always brave and sassy and beautiful.

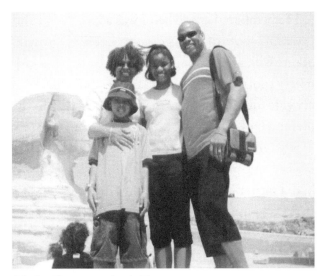

My family on vacation in Egypt

It was tough when I had to leave them to go back on duty. But there's something about me, I can easily turn it off and on. That way, I keep my focus on what I'm doing at the present time. It saved me from missing them too much.

Watching my kids grow up and mature gives me so much joy—to see them becoming more responsible, winning at sporting events. Tiyauna, who's 18 now, is captain of her high school basketball team, and it's good to see her showing leadership and taking control.

Harvey's 14, and I love to watch him play football. There's no better feeling in the world.

He's sensitive. If he feels like he can give something to someone in dire need, he'll do it—he'll try to help.

That's the type of person he is. But up there on the football or basketball field, I can see how he hates to lose, and I say to myself, *Man, is that the same kid who'll give the shirt off his back to someone else in need?*

For me, seeing my kids grow up and develop is the most interesting thing there is.

Last year I took my daughter to the debutante ball in Chicago, where they have sororities for teenagers. It's kind of an old-fashioned way for girls to get ready to step into society. Mostly it's the parents who decide they want their daughters to take part.

I remembered how when I was a kid, I was an escort to a girl going to a debutante ball, and I thought it would be a pretty cool thing for Tiyauna to do. So my wife found a sorority that was organizing a ball.

She felt like a bride that night, and I wore my marine uniform and we had a father-daughter dance. I don't think any man could have been more proud of his daughter than I was of her.

I didn't have that with my parents growing up, but now that I'm a parent, my kids and I talk all the time and it's great. My daughter talks to me in the middle of the night if something's on her mind, and if Harvey V is having a bad hair day he'll say: "Dad, let's talk."

It's great to communicate with my kids, and I value and treasure my relationship with them. I would give anything for them to have happiness and success.

It's your life, your world, so dig deep and take control of it before it's too late.

I figure it like this: A girl needs her father at that time in her life, to protect her and support her and tell her he's proud of her. Hell, if you don't tell her, how's she gonna know?

To me, what matters with my kids is just the everyday stuff. Just sitting and talking, playing PlayStation with my son, who gets all the cheat codes off the Internet and shows me how it's done, having good long chats with my daughter about what's going on in her life.

Sometimes you have to suck it up with teens, but you never stop supporting them. I remember how I had in mind that Tiyauna would become a medical doctor. I was eating breakfast in Los Angeles with her a year ago when she told me she wanted to major in psychology, not medicine. And even though I was really looking forward to her becoming a medical doctor, I looked at her and smiled and said: "You know, that's all right if that's what you want to do. Are you happy about it? Hey, I'll support you."

That's how it's got to be when you're a parent. You just get down in there and roll with the punches, but you never stop loving your kid and being there for them. They're depending on you, so what you gonna do, look the other way? That's not the kind of parent I aim to be.

Tiyauna's idea of fun is to relax with a book. She's like me; she'll grab four books and read them all at the same time. She's very mature for an 18-year-old and she's playing basketball at a college on the East Coast, where she plans to major in psychology.

I know that as a sportswoman Tiyauna has to take care of her body.

Women have to be especially conscious of how they take care of their muscles. I see how many women don't have the longevity in sports that some men have. Women tend to get more problems in their lower extremities than men.

So I've taught her to drink water, or if she's got a track meet with a lot of running, and she's been sweating a lot, to take a sports drink afterward and put the electrolytes back in her body so that she doesn't cramp. When she gets home she's learned to take a nice warm bath, relax and de-stress, with candles and music.

We all have to do that. I'm guilty myself of forgetting to relax or of not doing my stretches sometimes. Recently I played two rounds of golf with no stretching, and when I went running the next day, man, I felt sore.

If you want your kids to grow up fit and strong, the best way is to be involved in sports with them. My kids started out this way when they were 3 or 4 years old—just like I did with martial arts—and I'm glad they did. I believe that if you want a child to develop good hand-eye coordination, it's best to start early.

But it's never too late to make a difference. Not everyone can start playing sports at the age of 3. But you CAN start NOW. Even a little effort will make a lot of difference.

You've just got to take one step. That will make it easier to take another. And then when you've taken a few, you'll see that your whole life is changing, and man, you are on the road. Then the going gets easier.

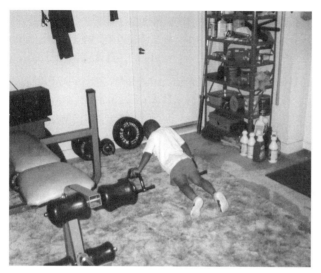

Harvey V when he was five years old, trying to copy Dad

My son, Harvey, goes to the gym every day now that he's 14, though when he's at home he'll relax by kicking a ball around the yard or playing his PlayStation. He never wanted to go to the gym with me, but now that I'm not there he goes on his own. He's a basketball player, and he's always said he wants to play for the NBA. I think he might do it, too.

He's got a lot of talent in track. When he was 12 he ran a 7-minute mile, and he flew down to Santa Monica especially to run against *Fit Club* contestants Kelly LeBrock and Gunnar Nelson—and beat them. Kelly had fallen off a horse just two weeks prior, but even so, Harvey ran well and I was proud.

For my kids, playing three sports a year has always been mandatory. The exercise helps to build health into their bodies, encourages them to socialize, and teaches them how to be a good sport, which means learning how to lose.

It's a tough lesson, but just like adults, kids need to learn that you can't ever win them all. You've always got to be a loser at some point, and the sooner you know that, the sooner you can start learning how to win in the biggest contest of all— with yourself.

That's why I DON'T accept excuses. Because it means you're losing in the contest against your own worse self, you're giving up the fight. And we're not in the fight to give up. We're in the fight to win.

So hold on to your motivators and keep moving, because that's how you will take control of your life.

I saw how it worked when my mom and dad split up. I was 8 years old, left at home taking care of my little brother. It was kind of scary, but I learned how to do everything and take care of us both. I learned how to win.

So I know the bottom line is: Parents make the best role models. Kids need validation and the example of good morals and good ethics. They need to know how to do the right thing before they hit their teens, when it's all about peer pressure. If you don't make money in the first ten years of your kid's life, you're way behind the eight ball.

I admit it, I'm a neat freak. I'd plan all the meals for the whole week on a Sunday, as well as get the yard work done, do the laundry, and change the sheets and towels. Sunday night was my relaxing time; after dinner when I'd finished the dishes I'd watch *60 Minutes* and then go mop the floors.

I always had a system, and when I was away from home, Sherry had to take everything on herself. And it was hard for her.

I've been training my kids to be responsible at home. Everything I

We're not in the fight to give up . . . we're in the fight to win.

My kids' mom, Sherry, ran track in high school, and she's always backed both of them in sports. She's done a great job with the kids.

It wasn't easy for Sherry when I started working on the TV show during weekends as well as working as a marine five days a week. When I was at home I was a hands-on dad, I ran my kids around, I always planned everything and executed it too.

used to do, they now do. They both do their own laundry; I've shown them how to sort it. Tiyuana does the dishes and the bathrooms; Harvey does the trash and the floors. When I started traveling more two years ago, I told him: "You're the man of the house now. Take care of your mom and your sister." He does the yard work and washes the cars. I've taught them both how to cook. I'm proud of

how well they know how to deal with life.

We have good times. Every year there's a Marine Ball, to commemorate the founding of the Marine Corps on November 10, 1775. I took Harvey and Tiyauna in 2006. It was their first time at the ball, and I knew it would be my last time on active duty as a serving marine. I thought it would be cool for them to see how the marines march in carrying a cake, and how there's a cake-cutting ceremony, with the first piece going to the youngest marine and the second piece going to the oldest, and the commandant's message read aloud at the ball.

It was an experience they'll never forget, and I was proud to have them with me.

Then at Christmas it was the kids who decided we needed some time to relax. "You're working so hard, Dad," they told me. "Let's have some down time. We want to go to Florida." So I packed up a small Christmas tree and we rented a villa for ten days.

I retired from the Marine Corps recently so that I could be there for Tiyauna and Harvey at an important time in their lives. I loved the marines, but kids' lives don't come back—you've got to catch them when you can. Harvey has started high school, which is a crucial time for him when I need to teach him how to be a man. And Tiyuana is starting college and I need to be around to help her.

I knew retiring would be a sacrifice, and it was hard to leave the Marine Corps after so many years, but I wanted to be there for my kids—for my daughter's first weeks at college, for my son's football games.

That's my motivator, my north star, the thing that never changes: my love for them. It's made me a better man and a better marine, and it's helped me to stay in shape mentally and physically.

Everyone has a motivator. So find yours and get moving, and you will notice the difference in your power and in your life. Don't just believe me. Try it.

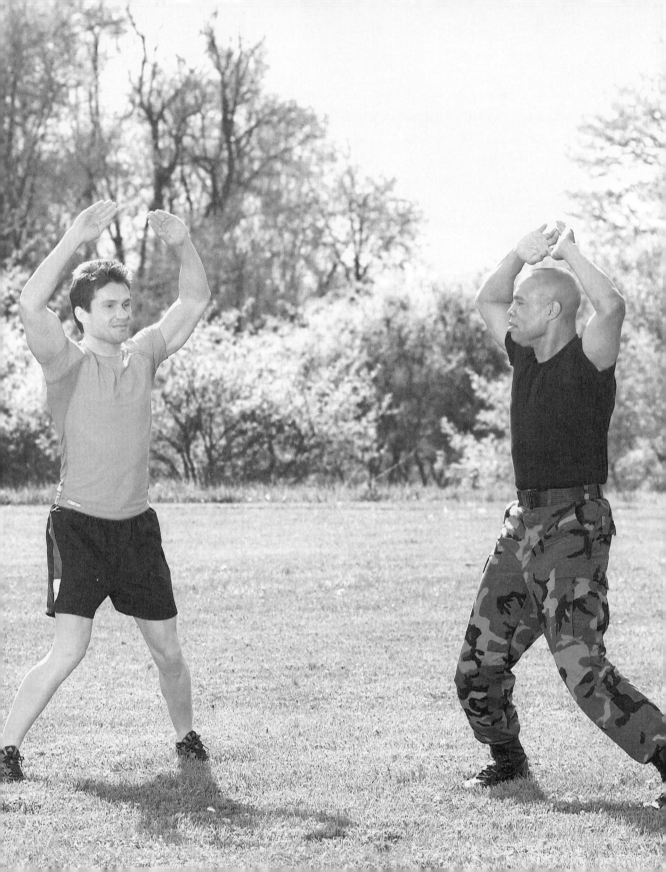

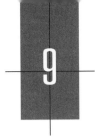

CLEAR YOUR HEAD WITH HARVEY

Okay, grasshoppers. We've come all this way and we're still in the fight against obesity and we're winning the war against whining and lazy-ass living. So go on, give yourself a prize and take some credit. If you are doing the exercises and taking care of your diet, you are on your way!

I'll be talking some more about diet later, but first I want to tell you about something else that will help you increase your motivation, sharpen your focus, and sort out your time management.

It can help you plan well with a purpose, and it keeps you going through the day, so we are making money right here by using this technique.

It's called tapping into your chi energy, your inner strength that you can use to get in the fight and keep motivated.

People often ask me what chi is. I was so young when I learned how to tap into it that it's hard for me to say. I just know it's there and I use it all the time. For me, it's using my energy reserves and to find my inner strength.

There are different ways of accessing your chi, through martial arts, Tai Chi, yoga, other Eastern philosophies. Hey, I'm a marine and I don't have time for soft crap. But this stuff does work and it can be a lifesaver. So check it out for yourself.

Different people have different ways of accessing chi but we've all got it there to use, so take my advice and tap into this river of energy running through you. Once you're in touch with it, man, ain't nothing can stop you from that point on. It is the key to that kingdom of healthy energy that will keep you going through thick and thin.

When you've found your chi, you can learn how to use it to your advantage.

I tap into mine through meditation.

Meditation is about calming down and letting go. Letting go of your thoughts and emotions, detaching, watching it all drift by. And then when you come back, you're sharp and focused and ready for the fight.

I could not live the high-octane life I do if not for meditation. It's something you can learn. My grandfather, Harvey Walden II, was the one who taught me.

I was just 3 or 4 years old when I started learning martial arts with my grandfather, and boy, was that an experience for a young kid. The style was jujitsu and aikido, and needless to say, I was the youngest in the group by far. Every morning my grandmother would iron our *gi*s (karate uniforms) and cook my grandfather and me the best breakfast a man could ask for. Then all day we would be training at the dojo in Chicago's South Side, near our home.

I could never understand why a kid had to spend all that time getting his ass kicked by these old guys and getting thrown around the mat like a rag doll. It was only as I got older that I realized it made me so damn tough, and when I started kickboxing, getting hit was never a problem for me.

All that time, though I didn't know it, it was also teaching me about control and balance and discipline.

Everyone can get angry and violent. It's easy to lose control. That's when your aggression takes over, your body floods with adrenaline, your mind clouds up with emotion and loses its way, you tense up and hit out, and that's when you can be badly hurt. That sure ain't the way of chi.

In martial arts there's another way. Go with the flow, roll with the punches.

You always finish off each martial arts training session with meditation. You calm your mind, which automatically calms your body, and it all works together to keep you in peak physical and mental shape.

No matter how bad I got kicked in the ass in those childhood years long ago at the dojo, it was always controlled. I was never really hurt. We always ended politely and we always sat down and meditated together afterward. We cleared our minds of aggression, anger, and hatred, and we went out clean.

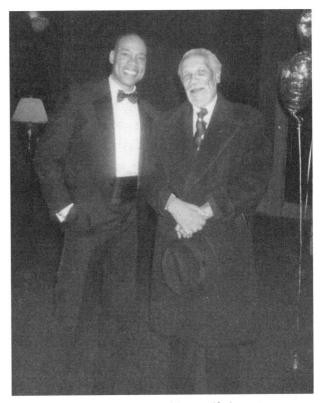

I love spending time with my noble grandfather

I HATED having to meditate at first, because it was such an uncomfortable position to sit in.

In aikido and jujitsu we do everything from our knees first. All our techniques are from our knees. But as a kid the very last thing you want is to be freakin' sitting on your damn knees at the end of a session.

I wasn't allowed to sit cross-legged. My grandfather took charge and he trained me good. It was the end of the day and I'd be the only one sitting there, and my grandfather, the guy who had been kicking my ass and throwing me around and making me mad in that dojo all freakin' day, used to make me sit there and meditate some more. Till HE decided I'd had enough.

The sun would be shining in through the window, and I was ready to go play.

But I couldn't get away. I had to do that doggone meditation.

I was always pissed off. And Grandfather would say: "You don't understand. Everything we did today was for a purpose. Now go over there and clear your mind and meditate. Close your eyes! Meditate!" So I had no choice. I had been humiliated all day and I carried on being humiliated.

But it worked. By the time I was 6 years old I was already a black belt.

You never need to put a time limit on a meditation session. Grandfather would just say that you knew for yourself when you were done.

I remember one time I tried it. I said: "I'm done."

He said: "You're not done."

So I said: "But you said I know when I'm done."

"You're not done," he said. End of conversation, and I still had to sit there just the same.

I was around 12 years old when the penny dropped, and I made a strong connection with the chi energy inside of me. Something happened in my family that I can't say too much about, and for once I lashed out. My grandfather came right over when he heard. His face was stern.

"Go meditate," he said.

It was a relief to get into that still place inside. I felt the anger ebbing away. I felt peace. I got it at that moment.

After that, no one had to tell me to meditate. I've done it on my own, most days, ever since. Because I NEVER want to lose control.

Meditating has helped me suck it up, roll with the punches, and focus, because inside myself, I'm calm.

And in high-stress situations, what you need is not to tense up but to stay just a little bit looser. To relax into the crisis, to keep your balance. It takes practice, but martial arts experts know that's a good way to live.

In martial arts, there's always a force to every counterforce. You use your opponent's own weight and aggression and fear against him. Grandfather told me never to use my fighting skills outside the dojo. Real martial arts people respect that rule.

Because martial arts has taught me how to relax and detach, it's saved my ass many times. Grandfather was right: Everything was for a purpose.

When you've had a good meditation session, that's when you can think properly. It's when I make my weekly plans and do my lists. I know that if

I'm eating well, exercising properly, and clearing my head out too, I'm gonna be a human dynamo and one hell of a guy.

You can be that same way. Diet, exercise, mind—they're all part of the same thing. They make you the best that you can be, and they keep you in the fight. That's our purpose.

Sometimes there are extreme situations where you really need that clear head.

just then a big gust of wind caught me and I started drifting my little light ass toward the trees.

It was my own fault. I'd been taking photos with a little camera, which you weren't supposed to do but we all did, and I hadn't noticed where I was going.

I realized that my focus had slipped for an instant. If I had been paying close attention, I could have gotten away from the trees as I fell, could have done something, but instead, because I

It's mind over matter, so suck it up, dig deep and find some chi.

I remember when I was jumping out of a C141 jet. It was a pretty cool job because when you went out the back of that bird, it was like that jet force just took you through the sky like a silver bullet or something, and I felt like I was in heaven just flying through the air.

So I was coming down. I was checking my altimeter, and everything looks good. I see the tree line. I was a pretty light jumper, I weighed maybe 165 pounds, and I got to the tree line and looked up and my chute looked good and I'm getting ready to land, when

was distracted by taking pictures, I got caught with the wind and was taken the wrong way.

And I thought, *Holy shit, I'm gonna crash and burn.*

I knew there was nothing I could do. So right there, falling through the sky, I turned to that discipline of meditation. I stilled my thinking and waited and let it drift. There was nothing else to do. I stayed calm and connected within my inner space just like I'd been made to do long ago by my grandfather.

That meant I was ready for whatever might happen.

So I broke through the big old top of the trees, and hit a tree, and crashed right through it, and a damn tree branch broke my fall, and I was down, hanging by my legs upside down on a tree branch. And I couldn't feel my legs. It felt like they were asleep.

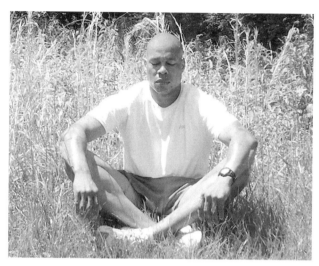

And for a minute there I was thinking, *Shit. I'm going to be paralyzed, I broke my damn legs,* and as I was thinking these thoughts, all the guys were standing around me freakin' laughing.

So I waited. And then, very slowly, I swung myself off that branch using my arms, unhooked my harness, dropped to the ground, brushed myself off, and strolled away.

I'd stayed relaxed. I'd rolled with the fall and yielded to the hit just like I'd been taught to do years before, and that's why I hadn't been injured.

I was completely unharmed.

Meditation clears your mind and it prepares you for all the things you've got to do next. I used to do it every evening, but now I just do it three or four times a week when I'm out running. For me it's so automatic that I don't even think about it. It's part of my life and always has been.

It's how I get a handle on everything I do, by clearing my mind. And if I go a couple of days without it, I sure feel the difference.

Relaxation is part of Harvey Walden's No Excuses! Fitness Workout. And there is NO excuse. We all need to relax.

If you can't work on your chi, or you don't know what it is, that's no problem. Just make sure you have some downtime in your busy schedule, and give your mind a break. It's part of stay-

LET IT ALL GO

There are a variety of activities you can practice to clear your mind and center yourself. Try these:

Breathe through your belly:

- Start by blowing out all the breath in your lungs.
- Focus on a point about two inches below your navel, in the center of your body. Inhale, imagining taking air all the way to that center and feeling your entire belly expand.
- Then breathe out slowly from that same place. Do ten of these breaths and let each exhalation relax your body a little more.

Meditation:

- Find a quiet, comfortable place, where you won't be distracted. Sit with your back straight and place your hands in a comfortable position.
- Focus on the sounds of nature, or quiet, soothing music if indoors. Allow your eyes to rest comfortably downward, gazing softly.
- Let your breathing become deep and rhythmic.

Let your muscles go:

- Start with three to five shoulder shrugs: Inhale while you tense your shoulders and lift them toward your ears; then exhale as you drop them and let yourself relax.

---

ing fit and healthy and in good shape, and meeting all of your commitments.

In my life, working 24/7 and flying three times a week, I make sure I take breaks. I'll go to a jazz café, or watch TV, or light a candle, or read. Sunday is when I hit the snooze button if I can. I make Sunday a day of rest.

It's important to take regular breaks. Hey, we all know you'll put yourself in the grave prematurely if you don't. And you don't want that. Not for your family, not for your loved ones, and not for yourself.

So remember. It's your life, you're in control. Clear your mind, find some peace, and then you'll start every day fresh and ready to go.

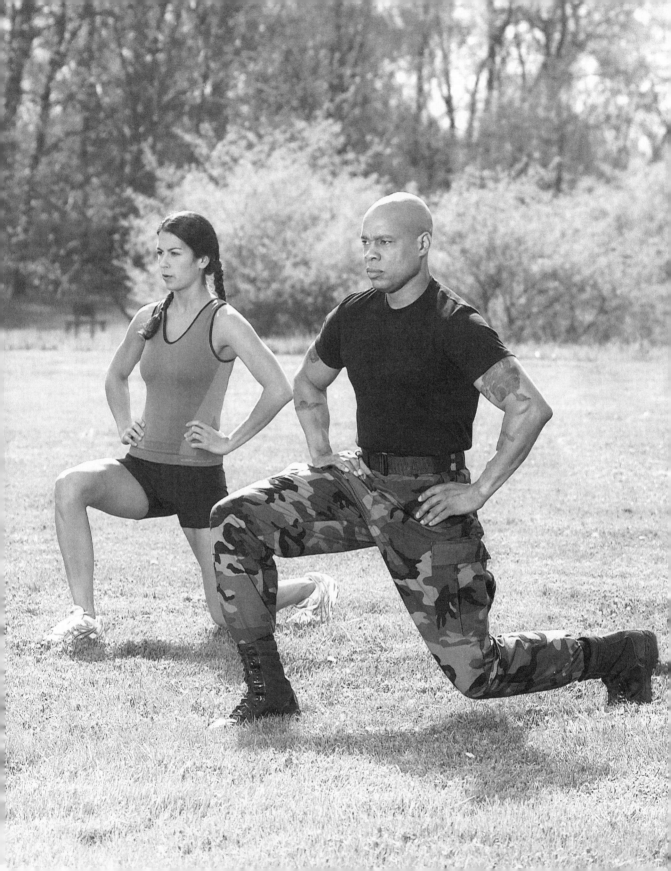

10

HARVEY'S NO EXCUSES! FIGHT THE FLAB FOOD PLAN

I have a rule of thumb about eating: No meal on your plate should be bigger than the size of your hand.

Nobody needs more than that at one sitting. Any more and I think you are into the badlands of overeating, by stuffing yourself unnecessarily and gorging your way to obesity.

So when you are loading your plate at home or out in a restaurant, you can always look at the palm of your hand, spread your fingers a little, and imagine that as the measure of your portions added together. For instance, if you are having a good old breast of grilled chicken, it should only be the size of the palm of your hand.

Keep inside those limits and you won't go wrong. My main No Excuses! message here is: DON'T CUT OUT, CUT DOWN.

I'm obsessed by portions. I truly believe that getting them right and doing positive sufficient exercise will lead you to controlled sensible weight loss and physical fitness that will make you feel good around the clock, because

ger than average, so the portion indicator works there, too. Your own body gives you the measure; you don't need nothing else.

As I say . . . NO excuses.

And I also accept that you, like me, can have five meals a day to keep the energy levels up. I eat five because I am always working out, on the go, and burning calories.

Your eyes should never be bigger than your belly.

your body will feel in shape and operate as it should.

Heck, most of us are lucky enough to know where our next meal is coming from, so we don't have to wolf down everything in sight.

Your eyes should never be bigger than your belly. Your eyes should take a good guide from your hand.

And if that don't get through to you, imagine Harvey's hand coming to clip you round the head for stepping out of line.

I have tried this myself all my life and it has done me well. If you're a big guy, then your hand is going to be big-

But those five do not have to be cooked meals. They can be healthy snacks, like green apples, which I personally can't get enough of, or other natural, unprocessed products.

I'll give you a list of items I swear by in Chapter 12.

In the meantime, let me give you an example of a day in my life and how I have come to understand what my body needs and how I achieve that balance, almost without thinking about it anymore.

After years of paying attention to my body, I have gotten to the stage where I know what my body needs and how I can compensate if my routine is changed through work or travel. I can balance things up.

My statistics hardly ever change. They are:

Height: 6 feet
Weight: 175 pounds
Chest: 44 inches
Waist: 32 inches
Neck: 15.5 inches
Boots: 12
Body fat: 7.8% (The average man's is between 15% and 17%. An elite athlete's is between 6% and 12%.)

I always wake up at 4:00 a.m. That's if I have had any sleep at all. Often I don't, because I have a lot of balls to juggle, between work and family life and a whole lot of traveling, but I manage to cope with loss of sleep because my body is in good shape and can handle that.

So I will lie there for a short while, thinking about the day ahead—although I always plan three days in advance so I have a shape to my life, which I need—focusing on my objectives.

Then I will have breakfast, which I think is vitally important to set yourself up for the next 24 hours of activity and provide the first intake of energy. In my case I have what I describe as five meals a day, although I am constantly eating.

With all meals and throughout the day, I'm drinking water. Just a glass with my food and a bottle in my hand all day long. To rehydrate is important, especially when you are exercising and running, so get into the habit of sipping water, not soda nor too much coffee and caffeine.

HARVEY-STYLE BREAKFAST:

Now I know I just said "not too much coffee or caffeine." Well, here is where the "not too much" part of that comes in. I always start my day with steaming hot black coffee. No milk. No sugar. I'd like to see you cut out those unnecessary fats and sugars.

I have a set of foods I rely on, but

it depends whether I am going to the gym first off, before work, or running.

If it's a gym day, I usually have some plain yogurt, some low-fat wheat bread, and a Nutri-Grain bar.

If I'm going running, I need something lighter, so I will settle for a coffee and then one of my favorite things on earth, a juicy green apple. That's enough if I am going to be running hard for an hour or so.

HARVEY'S APRÈS-MORNING-WORKOUT SNACK:

Some days I might be in the gym for two hours, so I'm quite hungry after that. When I'm at home I always have hard-boiled egg whites in my fridge. I prepare them at night a few days ahead of time, so I have some ready and have no excuses to reach for something else that might not be as good for me.

I cut out all the egg yolks and throw them in the trash. They aren't good for you because they are full of cholesterol. I'll eat only a small handful.

Or I might have a whole-wheat bagel with turkey bacon, which I really love. I don't have mayo or anything like that.

Any fruit in a small portion is good too.

HARVEY'S HOT HALF-HOUR LUNCH:

This always tends to be my "heaviest" meal of the day because it probably revolves around some cooked meat, and I like to have the rest of the day to digest it properly and work it off.

I know what my body wants, and I tend to keep my meals to around 400 to 500 calories. I was tested recently and I know that my body burns 2,423 calories in resting energy expenditure. That's because I am fit and my body is functioning well.

I take it seriously so that's why I

get these things checked. You should too.

So what I like is some grilled chicken. I use my Foreman grill all the time. I can throw a chicken breast into it and seven minutes later it's ready.

I'll have it with a little spinach or steamed broccoli. I don't prepare or eat these vegetables with any butter.

Or I might have thrown some chicken and vegetables into a stockpot and boiled them up for a few hours on the cooker. Then I can have that in portions throughout the week.

Too many people just pick up TV dinners from the store and throw something in the microwave. You really have to be aware of what's in those babies.

I'd say get yourself a lesson in grilling. It's easy and much cleaner and means you are taking in much less fat, which is important.

Again, I have to say, it's the "P" word that I am reminded of.

I never, ever clean my plate. It annoys some people, but they just have to get used to it. I can't overeat these days, my body just rejects it.

Like many of us, I was first trained by my grandma to clean my plate, and I would get a telling off if I left food untouched.

But the first time I remember doing that as a young boy, I felt bloated and fat and tired afterward. I thought, *Heck, that's just too much food.*

So I had to work out a little ploy because I didn't want to get in trouble or upset my grandma because she only wanted to feed me well—just TOO well.

I realized that I could limit the amount I ate and still have an empty plate by secretly handing it under the table to our pet dog Zena to eat. She knew to keep quiet and hide beneath the tablecloth so I could slide her bits of food. In the end we were all happy. Grandma was pleased, Zena was happy, and I was well satisfied with my meal, without any bloating.

Grandma meant well. But I'm glad I didn't get into eating all that food she put before me. Perhaps parents can think of that today with child obesity on the rise: that they could cut down on their kids' portions a little and help them develop good eating habits.

HARVEY'S MID-AFTERNOON SNACK

(and snacks for all occasions):

I snack all the time. I'm constantly putting things in my mouth in between meals, but it's not candy or chips or anything fried. I will have some peanuts, all kinds of dried nuts, grapes, or another green apple. I can eat those all day long.

Pineapples are also a big favorite with me. There are many healthy snacks around, like traditional or trail mix. I like to carry a big bag of this around with me and eat just a bit at a time, not the whole bag! The pretzel-style mixture is good because there is very little fat and no sugar in the contents.

I also carry a bag of apples or raw carrots when I am traveling because I can eat a few while I'm waiting at the gate at an airport or even on the plane. We all know how hard it is to find nutritious food when you are on the go. That's where planning your week comes in handy just like we discussed in chapters 1, 2, and 9.

HARVEY WALDEN IV'S SALAD:

Salads are one of my favorite meals, something simple, like a chicken Caesar with very light dressing, always works for me. I also like to have something from the ocean. I like most fish, and especially seafood like shrimp, lobster, and crab, grilled with a few lightly cooked vegetables. Not too much seafood too often; moderation is important with your diet.

Oily fish are good for the omega oils, so that's great too. I will have steak on the odd occasion, grilled, but not too frequently. I'm a chicken and fish man generally, and they keep me true to my target intake.

When I do have a meal that consists of meat, fish, or chicken and vegetables, I'll have a small green-leaf salad if I can. Sometimes that alone is enough with some egg whites. I use very little dressing usually, maybe just a light Italian or vinaigrette.

I try not to eat out much at all during the evening, but I often have to stay up late doing paperwork so I keep a bag of grapes with me to pick at. They're filling but good for you at the same time.

But it's okay to cheat too. Just the other day I was out and really got tempted to have some fried chicken. I made up for it the next day by getting back on track and working it off.

Like I've said, I don't mind the odd beer or two, even a cognac, and I do enjoy a big cigar. But these are once-in-a-while treats. I'm no angel and I'm far from perfect. So we all get tempted. The thing is to get back in the fight the very next day.

So, because I know what my body needs, I don't count the calories.

Some days if I am on a schedule where I can't get my meals in during the day, I have to eat in the evening. Some average Joe might see me in a restaurant at night eating some big plate of spaghetti or shrimp and say, "Look at that guy pigging out and he tells people what to do on TV."

What they don't know is that I'm not a hypocrite; it's just that I have probably come in under my ideal calorie intake for the day and I'm doing some balancing.

I'll still come up with the same range of calories, but not so evenly spread out during the day. It's all right to balance things out. And if you look at my pasta you won't find any fatty sauces or butter on it. Just a small sprinkling of Parmesan cheese and perhaps a few herbs for flavoring.

I don't really allow myself much in the way of sweet desserts. As I have already mentioned, I am a sucker for cheesecake, but it is the rare occasion when I have some and, even then, only a couple of forkfuls pass through my lips. I'm also quite partial to frozen yogurt. Again, a few bites will do it.

It's all about balance. I know that by feeding my body the right things, and not overeating, I've got a better chance of staying lean, healthy, and strong. That's a great basis for fitness, and it's a great basis for life, too.

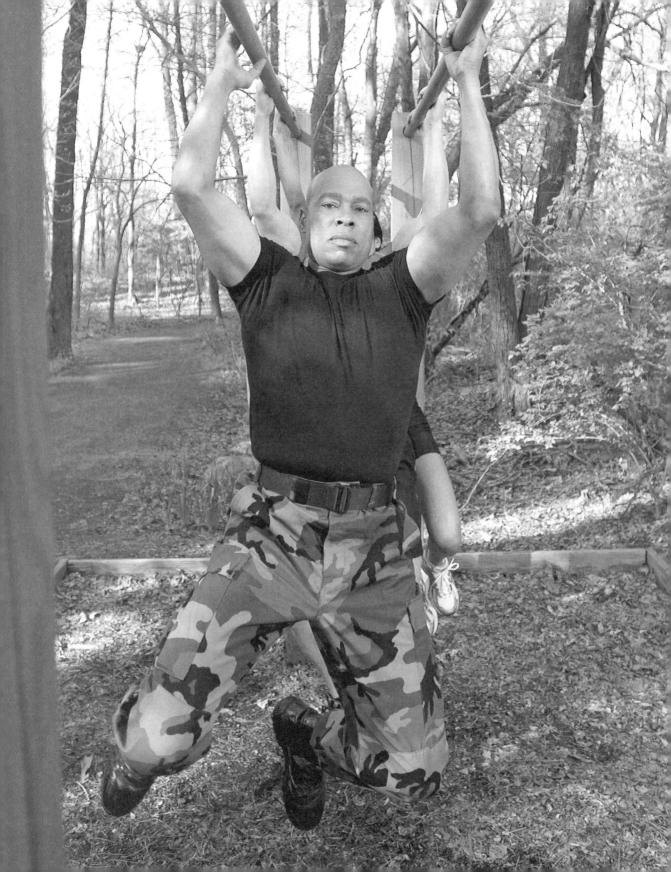

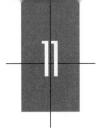

HOME COOKING WITH HARVEY

When I was 8 years old I taught myself to cook.

I had to. My mom and dad had been through a divorce, and there was my little brother, Milton, to take care of. And most times, nobody else was in the house but me, myself, and I.

I was the man. I had to step up to the plate and suck it up. Dad was away from home a lot, speeding off to work in his red Corvette or, in the evenings, to school. Whatever went on at home was all down to me.

Dad wasn't worried. He knew he could trust me. And he knew I'd get it together.

I did get it together. There had been a lot of pain in the family home and I blamed my mother for the rift between my parents. I thought my dad had done his best and I wanted to stand by him. So when the judge in that divorce court asked me which parent I chose to live with, I said my dad. I was a sassy kid and I'd made up my mind. I wanted to take good care of the house and my little brother and I wanted my dad to be proud of me. I wanted to prove I could do it.

My dad was always a hard worker, and when he wasn't working, he went to school as much as he could. I've lost count of the number of degrees he has. Even now that he's retired, instead of golfing and relaxing he's working on a thesis for another doctorate, in psychology this time.

When the going gets tough, my dad goes to school and gets a degree on the issue, to understand why it happened that way.

I'd grown up in what is now the ghetto of Chicago's South Side, in the 'hood between two ghetto turfs. We used to have local thugs pass through our neighborhood because we were the middle ground between rival gang territories: London Town Houses on one side of us, run by the Vice Lords, and Princeton Park on the other side, home of the Disciples or Folks.

Gangs were a very big issue in the area, but growing up, I never had any problems with either one of them, and actually went to school with members of both.

I guess that's why my father and grandfather took me into martial arts training so young: so that I would always be able to take care of myself. And I always could.

There were drive-bys where we lived too. I remember seeing my buddy Chris get shot in a drive-by on the sidewalk right across the street from where I lived. I was maybe 15 years old at the time.

Strangely enough, the gangs never made trouble for our family. To me that was natural. I had my dad and my grandfather, and my godfather and godmother lived only a couple of blocks away. Quite frequently we would go over for dinner.

My godfather was my uncle Milton's father, and damn, did I have respect for him. I would go over just to shoot the shit with him because he was such a tough guy. We called him the Godfather, and he lived up to every bit of his name, with tattoos up and down his arms, his ear pierced, and an interest in guns. And what did I become? A tattoo-wearing marine, and yes, I had my ear pierced before I joined the Corps.

Even the Godfather's dogs were mean as hell. He had Dobermans and a Great Dane, and those dogs were some mean suckers to most people, although I loved them. The Great Dane was called Peaches, and she used to let me ride her in the backyard, which was the coolest thing. One of the Dobes was called Slugger, and when the two of them got together and Peaches had fifteen pups, you best believe I used to sleep with each one of those babies in turn.

The Godfather kept his house shiny clean, and his grass looked like something you would play the Masters Golf Tournament on. So when one of the local thugs rode a bike through his grass, burning rubber and making fun of him, the Godfather wasn't taking it. He waited for the thug to come back, stepped out from around the garage, grabbed the bike seat, and just tore that kid's ass up. The gangs used to wear hats back in those days, turned to the side to represent their gang, and he snatched the hat off his head and spanked him with that too.

The kid never came back. I thought I might catch some flak about it at school, but I never did.

I never joined a gang. As a young kid, I had way too much on my plate to even think about running with gangs.

I was always close to my dad. Even before the divorce, he was always into cars, and when I wasn't at the dojo getting my ass kicked, I was at the racetrack watching him and my uncle Milton race.

I spent a lot of time in the garage with them as well, watching them work on their cars, and when Dad would go away I would copy what he just did on the car without him knowing. To this day I don't think he knows that I could probably take an engine apart blindfolded.

When I was 6 years old, we moved to a bigger house, farther away from my grandparents. Now, for the first time, my dad had the space he wanted for cars. I had five go-carts, especially made for me and very fast.

Of course he would always race me on the track and win. My cousin Randy and I would battle every weekend: As far as I was concerned we were the best drivers on the South Side of Chicago. The winners would go back and forth, of course, because we both were good enough to know how to keep anyone from passing once you had the lead.

As my little brother, Milton, got older he raced as well, and boy, was the

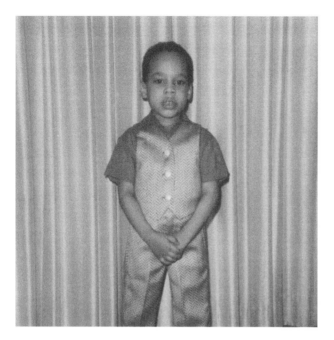

had to learn rather quickly, and thank God I started off in a healthy way. If I hadn't, who knows where I would be right now?

Because I had to learn how to sew and do other chores at a young age, it's made me more independent today. I do my own laundry, cleaning, cooking, and sewing. I really freaked out my *Celebrity Fit Club* wardrobe stylist one day when I was shining my own shoes. What she didn't know was that I used to shine my dad's shoes as a young kid well before I joined the marines.

I don't know why I started cooking steamed rice, vegetables, and spaghetti back then. And I'm still not sure how I learned to do it. I guess I just tried different ways until I found one that worked.

I would boil a pot of water and use a spaghetti strainer to put over the top of the pot, cover that, and then steam my rice and veggies.

That was mostly what Milton and I ate, and although my little brother

competition tough for him. Randy and I would wear his ass out so bad I felt sorry for the little guy. Needless to say, through all the fun I was having as a kid, having black belts in martial arts, riding go-carts, and hanging out having fun with my dad and family, I was still affected by the heartbreaking divorce.

That was the turning point for me as a kid. Now for the first time, I was really forced to take charge of the household. So who had to make sure we had dinner on the table and that the house was clean? You guessed it. Little old me. I must have gotten tired of it at the time, he tells me now that it's me who's made him the man he is today. So I must have been doing something right.

We did have other meals every so often, but steamed veggies and spaghetti was our standard dinner—maybe because I didn't know a whole lot else about cooking.

Of course, my favorite was peanut-butter sandwiches. Lord help you if you missed a corner of my bread and didn't cover it with some peanut butter.

Looking back, it wasn't a bad diet. Although it was a little bland and tasteless, the vegetables gave us some of the fiber, minerals, and vitamins we needed, and the spaghetti or rice gave us the carbs, and we got our protein and fat from the peanut butter. We didn't have much soda or sweets, nor hard, soft, or trans fats, nor hidden sodium or sugar—all those things that make you unhealthy, if they don't destroy you first.

I've taught my own kids how to cook, so that they're good to go and can face the big wide world without having to live on prepackaged foods full of additives. They know how to make stir fry, quick meals, and salads. And of course they know how to make

the Harvey Walden IV patented special: steamed vegetables and spaghetti, though I don't think they'll be eating it very often.

I was always pretty good at sports as a young kid, especially basketball and football. When I visited my mom on weekends, we would play football on the football field in the local stadium complex. I still don't know how we kept from getting arrested, because we literally cut a hole in the fence in one of the corners of the gate and would play full-contact football on the same field that all the high school teams played on.

How we got the equipment was another story. Our parents bought some of the gear, and some of the high school kids played high school ball, so we got knee pads and other items from them.

Of course, I was the youngest of all these guys, so damn, if I didn't take a beating most games. Again, I guess it paid off because I made the varsity high school team in my second year and turned out to be a pretty damn good player, playing semi-pro football as well, and I wasn't bad on track. In the end, I was voted the most athletic student in my high school.

My dad really tried his best to make sure Milton and I grew up as normal kids, even though there was so much drama going on in our lives.

I never thought I had it tough. I just sucked it up and enjoyed my life: winning in sports, winning in martial arts, riding go-carts, doing the best I could at home. My dad always told me he was proud of me and I knew that was true.

Now, looking back, I realize that nobody has it easy. Every person on this planet has their own personal problems, private just to them.

I work with celebrities, I work in TV, and I know that from Hollywood all the way to heaven, NO ONE is immune to problems.

We all have issues. Rich or poor, black or white, young or old, it makes no difference. You can't change the cards life deals you. That's your hand and you gotta play it.

But HOW you play it is up to you.

You might say it's too hard. Maybe life has dealt you a real bad hand. But I know that even in really bad times, there's usually something you can do. And taking care of yourself is a good start.

Fitness has always gotten me through, and I've helped many other people through fitness as well.

One hard thing for me, working on the TV show and still in the marines, was when I had to go back into military style. I had to snap the young marines into focus every now and then, because they looked at me on TV and thought, *This is Harvey*. They forgot that I was still First Sergeant Walden and I'd frigging rip their heads off if they had a bad hair day.

People also used to come up to me when I was in my military role and try to talk to me as though I was the Harvey they knew from TV. That could be difficult sometimes, but I just dealt with it.

I did have one bizarre celebrity experience once when I was walking past a Burger King in London and an overweight lady came rushing out holding a Whopper wrapper. She said, "You know, I watch your show and I think you're really motivating. Could you please sign this Whopper wrapper for me?"

She told me she thought that seeing me was a sign, and that she was going to stop eating Whoppers and start living properly. "And I'm gonna work out, I really am, you've inspired me," she said. She was even carrying a pen, and I signed her Whopper wrapper for her and wished her well. I should have kept in touch with her to see if she's still rocking and rolling.

But sometimes it goes the other way. Once in a Tesco store in England, just after the episode aired where I'd had a big argument with Rik Waller, an old lady came up to me and started shouting. She said I was a mean-ass, and I shouldn't treat people that way, and if somebody's to like you. But if you can do some good in this world, that's worth having.

I still keep in touch with a lot of people back in Chicago, and when I talk to old high school friends and they tell me that this guy is dead, or that guy is in jail, he got life, it's really weird. I see that all the gang members, the ones that weren't doing much other than the wrong things, are either still doing it, or they're dead, or they're in jail. They just hadn't done enough work

You can't change the cards life deals you. That's your hand and you gotta play it.

unhealthy and they're not fit they had personal problems and I needed to get to the root of the problem.

And then she kicked me hard, right on my leg.

I was shocked, and didn't say anything. It was one of those moments when you don't know if you want to snatch her cane from her and wrap it around her throat, or give her a hug and a kiss and say, "Okay, have a great day."

I just got in my car and left. I thought, *Well, that's how it is: You win some, you lose some.* Not everyone's going on their own lives to pull out and move on, and so they're still stuck, and some of them are dead or dying.

I don't want to be stuck in any way. No, sir. And you shouldn't either. That's why taking care of yourself is important. Having goals. Keeping a fabulously fit, toned body that works as well as you can make it work. And cooking for yourself is a big part of helping your body work.

Home cooking is the healthy option, it's economical, and it's not hard. Hell, if an 8-year-old kid could manage it, I think you can.

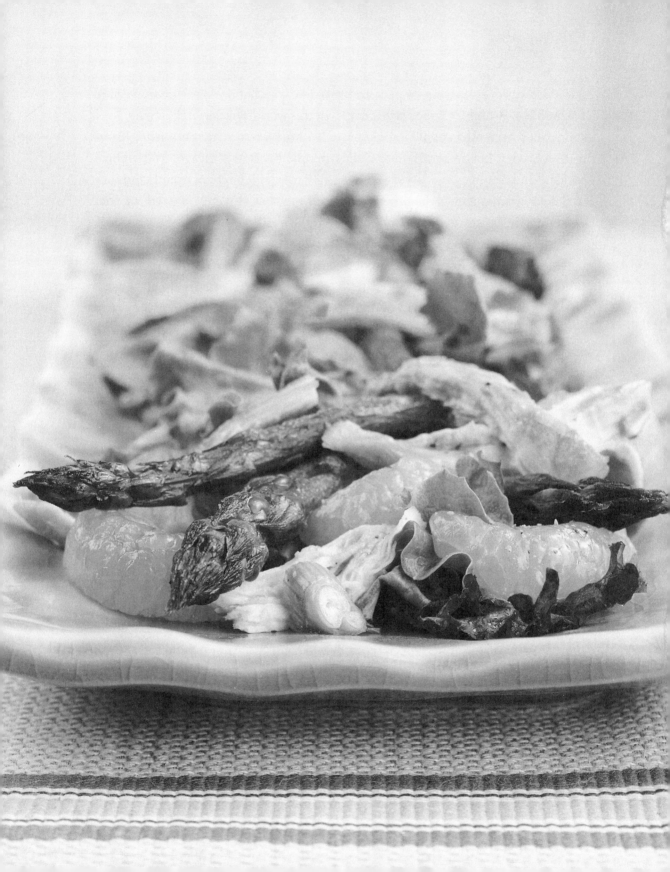

12

HARVEY WALDEN IV'S FIGHTING FIT GI FOOD PHILOSOPHY

As you know, my NO EXCUSES fitness plan is designed to help even the world's worst overweight couch potatoes get into the fight and change their lifestyles. That means YOU can extend your life too.

But while it's fine to go to war against fat and strive to improve your fitness, you're gonna have to do something about those bad refueling habits. Sitting around stuffing your face with pizza and fried chicken every day is the way to an early visit to the big man in the sky.

What you eat and how much you exercise go hand in hand. Working hard at building a better body is useless if you're filling it with trash as you go along.

I am in favor of a GI diet—no, not a military thing—based on the Glycemic Index, which is a term nutrition scientists use to measure the effects of carbohydrates on the body. It ranks carbs on a scale from 0 to 100 based on the extent to they raise blood sugar levels.

They discovered carbs behave differently and the GI index measures the speed with which they break down and how quickly they affect blood glucose levels. Glucose is the body's energy source—the fuel that powers the brain and fires the muscles and vital organs.

Eating low-GI carbs, ones that create only minimal changes in blood glucose and insulin levels, avoids instant "sugar highs" which, of course, are bad for us. These low-GI carbs provide long-term health benefits, like reducing the risk of heart disease and diabetes.

Following and understanding the measurements in the Index also provides us with a secret weapon in our war against weight. In short, foods that have a high GI are digested quickly and those with a low rating are absorbed slowly. Safe, slow, and steady is what we want. Just as in our workouts, remember those three little words: safe, slow, steady.

You'll get there in the end, believe me. No need to rush.

But that's NO EXCUSE to put off making this change in your eating habits. The sooner you get down to it, the better for you and your family.

I didn't go looking for a diet plan to follow. You read earlier about my typical daily intake of food and some of my favorite things to eat. I just moved toward the GI view of things naturally, really—just by listening to my body and responding to it.

Experts say that eating a lot of high-GI foods can be detrimental to your health because it pushes your body to extremes. This becomes even more true if you are already overweight and have a sedentary lifestyle. Of course, that won't be you for much longer under my watch!

Changing the habits of a lifetime and beginning to eat low-GI carbs will mean you will begin to balance your body by *slowly* feeding glucose into your bloodstream and keeping those energy levels on an even keel. You will feel fuller between meals. And you will avoid that dangerous sugar high.

Here's an example:

If you eat some cornflakes (GI 84) with some sugar (GI 100) sprinkled on top, that meal will be swiftly transformed into glucose, which will give your blood sugar level an almost instant "spike." You will get a rush of energy all at once. Bur pretty soon after, you will feel empty and want another hit of a high-carb food. And that's exactly what we DON'T want.

What we DO want is a slow release of energy. So by eating (and drinking) low-GI foodstuffs like traditional oatmeal (GI 51), which will break down slowly and feed into your bloodstream steadily and safely, you will avoid being "spiked" and feel fuller for longer.

Just one of the bad aspects of the sugar rush is that insulin is activated to extract sugar from the blood and store it immediately for use in the muscles . . . as FAT around the waist hips and thighs.

The bigger the spike, the more insulin is released, and suddenly you have fat deposited exactly where you don't want it and a deficiency of sugar, so you turn again to some sugary item to give you another high. These highs and lows must be avoided.

What I've always aimed at (without knowing it, in my early days) is a diet of low-GI foods, lean proteins such as fish and monosaturated/polyunsaturated fats such as olive oil.

The "Home of the Glycemic Index" is the Human Nutrition Unit, School of Molecular and Microbial Biosciences, University of Sydney, Australia. They also house the International GI Database and give this guidance:

- Low-GI diets help people lose and control weight
- Low-GI diets increase the body's sensitivity to insulin
- Low-GI carbs improve diabetes control
- Low-GI carbs reduce the risk of heart disease
- Low-GI carbs reduce blood cholesterol levels
- Low-GI carbs can help manage the symptoms of Polycystic Ovary Syndrome
- Low-GI carbs reduce hunger and keep you fuller longer
- Low-GI carbs prolong physical endurance
- Low-GI carbs help re-fuel carbohydrate stores after exercise

How do you switch to a low-GI diet? The GI experts in Sydney say the basic technique is to simply swap high-GI carbs for low-GI carbs.

The scientists, who form the prestigious GI Group, advise:

- Eat whole grain breakfast cereals based on oats, barley, and bran
- Eat breads with whole grains and stone-ground flour
- Eat fewer potatoes

- Enjoy all other types of fruit and vegetables
- Eat basmati or brown rice
- Eat whole grain pasta
- Eat whole grains like quinoa

- Eat plenty of salad vegetables with vinaigrette dressing

This is all underlined by a recent study from the Harvard School of

GLYCEMIC INDEX 101

The Glycemic Index (GI) ranks carbohydrates according to their effect on blood-sugar levels. Sugar in your blood is what gives you energy, and so we're programmed as human beings to crave it. A sudden high-sugar rush, as from high-GI foods, gives you a quick hit, making you feel more satisfied, more alert, even happier. But it doesn't last—and it's more likely to make you fat.

So it's time to get smart, beat the opposition, and go for the low GI. Low-GI foods keep your blood sugar properly topped up to the steady level you need for health. These foods will keep you satisfied and energized all the time. That way, you don't have to eat more than you need.

It's all about the blood-sugar level, grasshoppers, so take a look at these numbers and get used to

BAKED GOODS

Waffle 76
Bagel 72
White bread 70
Whole wheat bread 69
Bran muffin 60
Pumpernickel bread 41

CEREALS

Cornflakes 84
Cream of wheat (farina) 70
Shredded wheat 69

Old-fashioned (rolled) oats ..59
All-Bran™ 42

GRAINS

Instant rice 91
Millet 71
White rice 68
Brown rice 55

PASTA

Brown rice pasta 92
Boxed macaroni
    and cheese 64

Linguine* 46
White spaghetti* 41
Meat-filled ravioli* 39
Whole grain spaghetti 37
Fettuccine 32

LEGUMES

Canned pinto beans 45
Black-eyed peas 42
Chickpeas 33
Lima beans 32
Butter beans 31

Public Health, which indicated that the risks of diseases such as type 2 diabetes and coronary heart disease are strongly related to the GI of the overall diet.

In 1999, the World Health Organization (WHO) and Food and Agriculture Organization (FAO) recommended that people in industrialized countries base their diets on low-GI foods in

choosing the food that's right for you. I promise, if you stick with it, you'll feel healthier and you'll look better, too.

I've pulled together the GI ratings for some common foods to get you started. The lower the number, the better it is for you to eat. The only exception is that foods given in *italics* are okay to eat even though they have a high GI, because they're mostly fiber and water, so they have much less effect on blood sugar. Foods high in fat and calories have an asterisk (*), meaning you should avoid them except as an occasional treat. And remember—if you have a bad day, I want you to get right back in the fight afterwards.

DAIRY AND ICE CREAM

Ice cream 61
Sweetened fruit yogurt 33
Fat-free milk 32
Whole milk 27
Artificially sweetened
    yogurt 14

FRUITS

Watermelon 72
Banana 53
Orange 43
Grapes 43

Apple 36
Peach 28
Plum 24

VEGETABLES

Baked potato 85
French-fried potato 75
Carrot 71
Fresh mashed potato 70
Fresh corn 59
Green peas 48
Tomato 38

SNACKS

Pretzels 83
Corn chips 72
Popcorn 55
Potato chips* 54
Chocolate 49
Peanuts 14

order to prevent the most common diseases of affluence, such as coronary heart disease, diabetes, and obesity. For further information, go to www.glycemicindex.com.

Take a good, long look at that last paragraph. We've got an epidemic of obesity going on here, so get off that couch and get into shape . . . NO EXCUSES. So what about the protein and the fats?

If you are into your meat for your protein, then try to avoid those that are high in fat. Head for the supermarket case where the lean meat, fish, and poultry are. Look for cuts that are trimmed of fat or are skinless. Consider other sources of protein, too, like soy.

Foods like cheese, butter, and fatty meats are loaded with saturated fat. Worse still are processed foods like cookies and chips, which are full of trans fats or hydrogenated fats.

The best things to aim for are polyunsaturated fats, like most vegetable oils, or monosaturated fats, like oils from olives, rapeseed, and most nuts, and omega-3 fats in fish such as salmon.

Avoid salt wherever possible. I have to use it because I do a lot of running. But the general rule is to cut back where you can. It'll help your blood pressure.

Food can be fun, even when you are trying to lose weight. Promise yourself a really healthy, tasty treat as a reward for doing my NO EXCUSES Hot Half Hour Burn. Here are just a few examples; all are GI good and calorie low.

Some of the ingredients you will already have in your kitchen cupboards, and others you may have to find at the supermarket. Turn this to your advantage. You can walk there if it's not miles and miles away. Or you can park a mile away and walk the rest of the way to the store.

Or if you ride a bus or train, get off a few stops earlier, and power-walk the rest of the way. All I'm saying is to go the extra mile and introduce exercise at every level of your life.

Then fill up those bags with chicken and tuna and vegetables and carry them back. You'll be turning yourself into an efficient fat-burning machine, which is the way we want it.

Now you have the good foods you need and you burned an extra 1,000 calories getting it. You'll feel better already and proud of your achievement. Now reward yourself with some terrific chi-ow.

That's an order!

HARVEY'S NO EXCUSES LOW-GI RECIPES

Marine-ated Grilled Tuna

This one is perfect for après power-walking, when you get back so hungry you could eat a horse. I don't have any recipes for that, but this is much better for you anyway. So light and full of wholesome goodness, yet tasty too.

Ingredients

1 thick tuna steak

Pinch of salt and freshly ground black pepper

1 tablespoon light soy sauce

Zest and juice of 2 limes

¼ of a small red chili pepper, seeded and finely chopped

¼-inch piece of fresh ginger, peeled and finely chopped

Olive oil spray

Method

Place the tuna in a shallow dish and season with the salt and pepper.

Mix the soy sauce, lime zest and juice, chili pepper, and ginger in a small bowl and pour over the tuna. Leave to soak for 30 minutes.

Preheat a nonstick grill pan over medium-high heat and lightly coat with olive oil spray.

Place the tuna steak gently in the pan when it is very hot and cook quickly for 2 to 3 minutes on each side.

DON'T overcook.

Great with a small, green leaf salad, maybe with a touch of vinaigrette if you have done your exercises thoroughly.

Grilled Dill Chi Chi Salmon with Olive Sauce

Salmon is a great low-GI food because it's also a rich source of omega-3, a good fat high in antioxidants.

Ingredients

1 medium-sized salmon fillet

1 lemon

1 teaspoon of chopped fresh or ½ tsp dried dill, divided

4 or 5 black olives

A big pinch of fresh parsley

A speck of salt (optional)

½ cup plain yogurt

Method

Preheat the broiler to medium high.

Line a pan that will fit under your broiler with foil. Place the fillet in it.

Squeeze a little lemon on the fish and then sprinkle half the dill on it.

Place in the broiler for 3 minutes.

Turn the fillet over and coat the other side with the remainder of the lemon and dill.

Broil for 3 more minutes and remove.

Chop the olives and parsley into small pieces, add the salt, and mix all into the yogurt. Spoon the sauce over the salmon and serve.

Harvey's Hot to Trot Apricot Turkey

This is a tender, moist turkey breast, packed with dried apricots for a feast full of flavor.

Ingredients

1 palm-sized piece of turkey breast

Zest of ¼ of an orange, chopped

2 ounces dried apricots, chopped

¼ cup plain yogurt

½ teaspoon each cumin, turmeric, coriander

½ clove of garlic

A pinch of salt and freshly ground black pepper

Method

Preheat the oven to 375° F and line a small baking pan with foil.

Slice the turkey breast horizontally to make two thin slices.

Pat orange rind, salt, and pepper onto one side of each slice.

Sprinkle half the dried apricots on top of each slice.

Roll up the turkey slices fruit side in, and secure with a toothpick. Place the turkey in the baking pan.

Mix the yogurt, spices, and garlic in a small bowl and brush onto the rolled breasts.

Bake for about 30 minutes or until cooked through.

Serve with basmati rice and steamed broccoli.

Healthy Heart Harvey-Style Broccoli and Cauliflower Salad

I know this one doesn't sound attractive to the palate, but believe me, it is flavorsome and so, so healthy. So give it a chance. Add a small amount of meat to it, keep it chilled, and you can have portions ready for a swift meal for three days. Try this with grilled chicken or turkey breast, or even lean ham!

Ingredients

9 ounces broccoli, cut into florets

1 small cauliflower, cut into florets

½ small red onion, chopped

2 tablespoons extra virgin olive oil

4 teaspoons lemon juice

1 tablespoon Dijon mustard

1 teaspoon chopped fresh tarragon

Pinch of salt and freshly ground black pepper

Method

Steam the broccoli and cauliflower for about 5 minutes. Do not overcook!

Place them in a big bowl, and stir in the onion, olive oil, lemon juice, mustard, tarragon, salt, and pepper. Let sit for a few minutes to marine-ate.

Serve on its own, or with a small amount of lean meat.

Gut-Reducing Lemon and Parsley Chicken

These chicken parcels have an exciting tang and make a great healthy dish at any time of the year.

Ingredients

¼ of a lemon

1 clove of garlic, thinly sliced

Large pinch of fresh parsley, chopped

A pinch of salt and freshly ground pepper

1 palm-sized chicken breast

1 teaspoon olive oil

Method

Preheat the oven to 375° F.

Remove the pulp from the lemon and dice into small pieces.

Mix the garlic, parsley, lemon, salt, and pepper in a small bowl.

Carefully cut a pocket into the breast lengthwise. Try not to slice it all the way through or the filling will fall out.

Stuff the breast with a generous helping of the lemon mixture, and secure the pocket with a toothpick.

Place the breast in a baking pan, cover with foil, and bake for 30 minutes. Then remove the foil and cook for a further 5 minutes to brown the meat.

Serve with a crisp green salad.

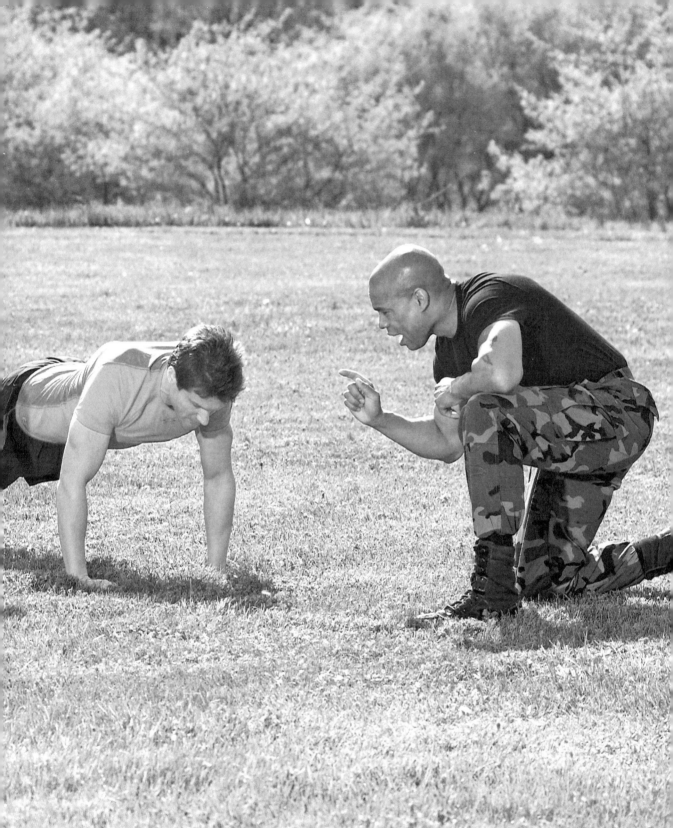

13

HARVEY'S Q&A

I get asked questions wherever I go, not only about fitness but problems relating to the human condition too.

People have seen me on *Celebrity Fit Club* and maybe they've seen my fitness DVDs and my own Web site.

I'll answer at any time, any place, because I think we're all in this together and let's help each other if we can. Surely it's to the benefit of us all, right?

It don't cost nuthin' after all.

These are the kind of questions I get hit with:

Q: I'm really worried I will never again have the great body I had when I was 21. I'm now 31 and my size is creeping up every year. I've tried diets and aerobics and nothing works. I work long hours at a desk and when I get home my husband says I'm fine and sexy. But I don't feel fine. What can I do?

A: That's a bowl of bullshine. I'm 40 and I'm training for America. I work with 70- and 80-year-olds who make me feel ashamed. And you should be too. Get it straight: Take in fewer calories than you are going to burn doing your daily stuff and exercise and you will see an early improvement.

Start by grabbing your old man and take him power-walking. It won't hurt you and you'll both feel great. Then you'll probably burn some fun calories off later.

Record your weight and weigh yourself every Saturday or Sunday, and then you'll feel happy if you've kept yourself honest and shed some pounds.

If not, you've got the next week to get back on track.

Q: What's the best kind of exercise to prevent brittle bone disease? I'm a 52-year-old woman and my mom, who's 84, is crippled with osteoporosis. I'm fit and well and I don't want it happening to me. What should I do?

A: You're right to think about this. We have to be aware of genetics and look at our parents for clues about how we might travel in later life. We have to be honest with ourselves and then we can work with what we've got.

First thing is to see your family doctor and have a talk about it.

I'm quite a fan of water aerobics because it's a low-impact activity, yet an exercise that is so good for many people who aren't fully fit or are a little delicate. But don't underestimate what a good workout you get from the pool. It'll get your heart rate up and burn the calories. Even gentle swimming is good for every muscle group and cardiovascular maintenance.

Q: I'm an extremely busy 36-year-old male who has little time to exercise and I've put on about 20 pounds in the past couple of years. Do you have any suggestions on how I can lose weight quickly and efficiently?

A: I could come around there and whup your ass. That would get you moving whatever time of day it is. People always come up with this trash.

Look, it's your life and you have to get it in perspective. Do you want to be fat and prematurely dead or do you want to get up half an hour earlier, do some power-walking around the block, walk to the station rather than take your car to work, and walk up the stairs?

It's obvious. But if you want to check out early . . .

Q: I'm 15 and I've always loved swimming and want to be on the school team, but I'm scared of getting those gross big shoulders like you see on Olympic girl swimmers. Is there any way I can train and still stay cute?

A: You shouldn't worry. Your shoulders won't bulge massively through training for the swim squad. In fact your upper body will be beautifully honed and toned and you'll look great in the mirror—and to boys. You'll also glow with good health and that's an attractive feature. Sounds good, huh? Get swimming!

Q: After having a baby 18 months ago my waist has spread and so has my ass and I've put on 30 pounds. It's horrible. I thought it would all go back to normal on its own, but it hasn't. Can you help?

A: I'm working with a girl right now who was 70 pounds overweight when she had a baby. We've gotten her down from a size 18 to a 4 in a few months, and all we did was work on the cardio and diet front. We all know that cosmetic surgery is the wrong way to go. It's lazy and it's intrusive and there's no need for it in most weight situations.

My girl stuck to her guns even though it seemed a long haul. We started with portion control—she'd gotten used to eating for two, I guess—and then we worked on her exercise, making sure more calories went out than were taken in.

And then, just running around after a baby is going to give you a good work out. Start sensibly and ask your doctor to monitor your progress.

Q: I'm 24, but I'm already suffering from man boobs, or "moobs." They're not huge yet, but they do seem to have been steadily developing over the last few years. I'm considering having liposuction on them because I've heard you can get really good results quickly. But my girlfriend is pleading with me to try exercise first as she's worried about the dangers of surgery. I'm not a big fan of exercise though, so wondered if there were any shortcuts you could suggest.

A: Come on, man! What have you been putting in your coffee? Listen to your girlfriend. She seems to be the one with all the brains.

Okay, genius. Let's say you have the lipo, the quick fix. But what does lipo do for your damn laziness about exercise and lack of self-discipline with your diet? You don't have to be a rocket scientist to pull the answer out of your fat skull to that question:

NOTHING! YOU GET THE FAT BOOBS AGAIN BECAUSE YOU DO NOT EAT RIGHT AND EXERCISE!

There is no shortcut. Get your diet fixed and get some workout action. Focus on hitting the chest exercises more with bench presses, push-ups, dumbbell work and close hand/ diamond push-ups (press-ups).

Trust me: Don't take the path of least resistance when it comes to your health, my friend. You only have one shot at life. Not of us is perfect, but God has given us the tools to get the job done. And you just might just have a little more stamina to please that great girl who cares about you. . . .

Q: I used to be really fit, but after a long illness I'm now out of shape. I'm a 28-year-old female, and when I started going to the gym again, I went hell-for-leather. But I pulled muscles and made myself sick again. Can you give me some advice on how to build up slowly so that I can get my fitness and figure back?

A: Grasshopper, let me first say: DON'T RUSH IT. You will never be able to come back after an illness, especially a long one, and pick up right where you left off.

It is difficult, but I can tell you are determined. Believe me, it will happen. What you have to do is be motivated by the fact that you WILL in time get it all back.

Start slow and with lighter weights or levels. Focus on your form and doing the exercises with quality and good breathing. Take it steady and very, very gradually lift those levels. Soon you will see the improvement and that will be further motivation.

Just make sure you do a good warm-up and cooldown and stretch afterwards. That's really important.

Q: I'm fairly happy with my size 10 figure, but I have these awful saddlebags just underneath my butt that I hate. It makes wearing tight pants a big no-no, and I hate wearing thongs. What exercise can I do to get rid of them?

A: Saddlebags underneath your butt? Just when I thought I'd heard it all.

I want you to get on a stationary bike for a 30-minute workout. After you ride with those saddlebags into the sunset like a female John Wayne, then try this lower body workout.

Do leg presses, leg curls, and walking lunges (they are explained earlier in this book) for 4 sets of 12 reps with light weights, and no more than a 2-minute break in between sets. Keep your movements smooth and controlled. If your form is sacrificed, then the weight is too much. Do these three times a week.

Cycle four or five times a week. But after a few weeks, switch up the cardio work and jump on a Stairmaster or stepper.

Q: I've been going to the gym three times a week for the past four months and I'm bored out of my mind. I try to do 30 minutes of weights followed by 30 minutes on the cross-trainer. I've been told that you need to change your routine every six weeks, otherwise it won't do anything for you—but I don't see how I can change it. Help!

A: Come on, grasshopper. Are you working out on the jungle gym at McDonald's? First off, buy yourself some new workout clothes and take a couple of days off from the gym.

No more than a few days, because you really sound demotivated, and I'm not there in your face to jump-start you. But I also don't expect you to be feeding your face with junk food over those two days!

I want you to pick up a women's fitness magazine and thumb through it for inspiration. Next, plan a new workout. Go to your gym, and this time hit the cardio first for 15 minutes. Feel free to take your new magazine and read it while riding the bike.

Also take your MP3 player. If you are still working out to the Bee Gees and *Saturday Night Fever*, it's time to download some new tracks, grasshopper.

After the 15 minutes, jump on the cross trainer for another 15. Check your intensity level to make sure you aren't sticking with the same level until the cows come home.

After that, pick a machine in the gym for each body part. Arms, chest, back, shoulders, legs, and abs for 3 sets.

Keep an exercise diary (I show you how to do that in Chapter 3) and change up the order after two weeks. Imagine that, grasshopper ... We have changed your routine.

NOW DROP DOWN AND GIVE ME 20!

Q: I started a diet about a month ago. I have been doing about 6 miles on an exercise bike and I am not losing any weight. I'm eating pasta and rice and some grilled meat, but I'm still not losing any pounds from around my stomach, which is what I want.

A: Come on, man, you're having a major malfunction with your diet. If you want to lose weight, you simply have to burn more than you take in. You seem to be putting in way too many calories. Start with getting a nutritionist or your doctor to look at your diet. I'm willing to bet you are screwing it up big time!

I've said it a million times ... watch your portion control: make it reasonable, like the size of the palm of your hand.

And make sure your exercise is quality exercise, not like a stroll in the park. Watch that heart rate to make sure you are pushing through without overdoing it, and change the routine every so often. But above all, stay in the fight!

Q: My arms are starting to wobble and there is no way I want to get bat wings. What can I do to tone them up? I'm a 35-year-old female.

A: No, we sure don't want you to have bat or bingo wings wobbling around, do we? I take it you are doing some cardio work, more than just a walk to the station?

You have to hit the gym and do your cardio work, and this weight training session 3 times a week for 4 sets of 12 to 15 reps:

E-Z curl bar, tricep pushdowns, alternate dumbbell curls, and dumbbell kickbacks (see Chapter 7 in this book, but if in doubt, ask a trainer at the gym).

In the morning when you wake up, drop down and knock out a couple of sets of press-ups. It goes like this: Before you brush your fangs, do one set with your hands close together for diamond or tricep press-ups, then a set with your hands in a normal position, about shoulder width apart. Then brush your fangs and wobble on the floor for another set.

In a few weeks your wobbly wings should be tight and trim like an anorexic turkey.

Q: I'm proud of my shapely size 12 body. I'd like to tone up a bit, but I don't want my breasts to get smaller. What exercises should I try, and what should I avoid?

A: WOW! You put way too much sugar on your corn flakes this morning. I would like to know this TOP SECRET workout that miraculously performs breast reductions while you sweat your butt off in the gym.

Don't get me wrong. Will you lose some size in your breasts when you start working out? Yes, if you are FAT and OVERWEIGHT! You will obviously lose some size due to the fat loss your entire body will shed from the proper diet and exercise.

If you are making money with those two elements, then what you lose will be what you needed to lose. You will not drop several cup sizes because you are a stud in the gym, so get the heck back in there and work it out.

You have to wake up pretty early in the morning to even think about pulling something like that on me, young lady. NO EXCUSES.

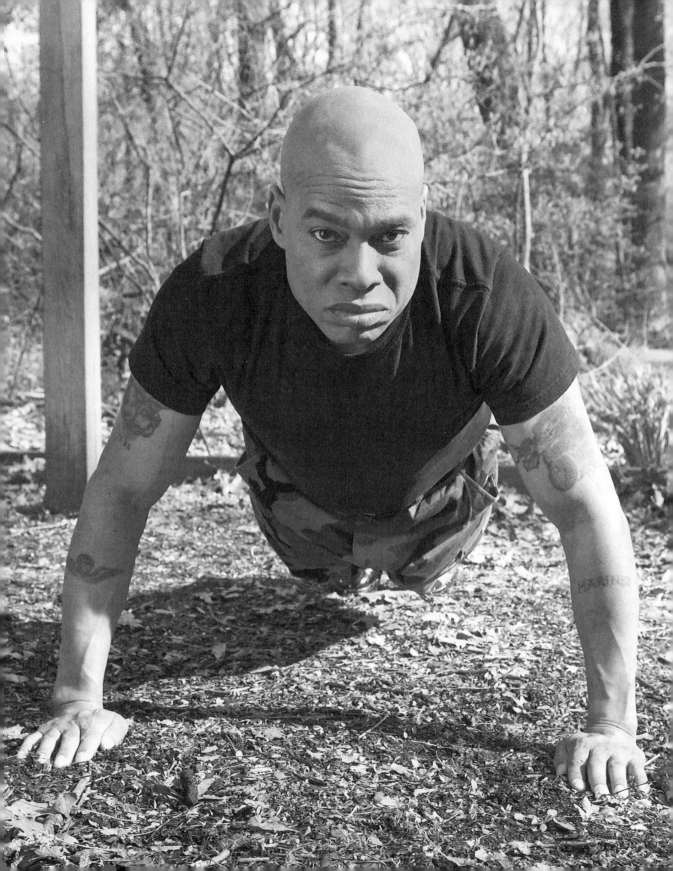

14

A NEW START

So here I am, 40 years old, standing in the drill yard in Fort Knox.

It's a warm evening. There's no one much around. The shadows are lengthening, and far away the road stretches out to the horizon. Soon I'll be gone from this place.

I retired from the marines last month. What will the future bring? I don't know.

There's only one way to find out: to step forward and live it.

I've trained thousands of young marines. I saw them turn from kids into men. Able to hold their own in extreme situations, to go out into the unknown and come back with honor. Willing to pay the price to serve their country. The few, the proud. That was us.

I remember those squad bays. I remember the sunshine mornings, the dramas and contests. The kids who made it—and the ones who didn't. The tears and the triumphs.

It was a good life. The marines have taught me more than I can repay. I'm glad I served.

But change comes to everyone. You can't escape. Sometimes you've got to get out of that comfort zone and meet the next challenge.

And I know that when it's time to move, there's only one thing to do: get off your butt and get going.

I'm on a new mission now. I'm in the fight against obesity with all my readers, and I aim to win.

People need to know that obesity CAN be solved, that we CAN live fit and healthy lives. When your body is well-tuned, it changes everything.

So I'm getting focused. And I want you to get focused too.

I wake up pretty much every day at 4:00 a.m. and get up about 30 minutes later after thinking about the day ahead.

Each and every day I'm going to exercise, whether it's in the gym or outside for a run.

You might say: "Well, that's okay for him. It's not so easy for the rest of us."

I'll let you in on a secret here.

I have as much difficulty as you getting up and motivating myself. I'm by no means perfect. This isn't easy for any of us.

Sometimes, rarely, I admit, I might have stayed up late socializing.

That means I have to push myself harder the next day to regain the lost ground. Make up for stepping back a few paces.

It's a motivator.

Throughout this book I've shared with you a number of things I say to others to push them on. What I'll say to you now is that the reason that I know these thoughts help is because I say these same things to myself to push me on.

If I have one mantra it would be: STAY IN THE FIGHT.

This works on so many levels.

It could be you are having a tough time exercising, or at work, or in your private life. We all go there, believe me. None of us escapes.

But I truly believe that by staying in the fight you will eventually win. I know it's true, because I've done it all my life. It works.

So I will say to myself: STAY IN THE FIGHT.

And then I will add: Don't give in because that's what they want.

That helps me carry on even when it's tough. When you carry on, you DO win. It's your life, and you are in control.

acknowledgments

This book would have never been written without the support of my immediate family and friends, who I would like to thank for all their support and love through it all. Lord knows I can be one tough cookie to deal with, and my family has really been there to see me through it all. Especially my son and daughter, Harvey V and Tiyauna Denise, who had to sacrifice some weeks when I had to work and not be home for those times when they really needed me. I love you two very much and am very proud to be your dad. May you have all the blessings and success that life can give you. Lord knows you deserve it after living a life of Boot Camp with me.

Of course, my thanks go to Gordon and James Poole from the Gordon Poole Agency. What took you two so long to find me after all those agents I had in the past? Thank God you did, and James, you really ROCK! It really is my privilege, honor, and pleasure to call you my agent and manager, but more importantly, my friend. Thanks for all your hard work and loyalty through it all. It really means a lot.

My Marines and the Corps that I have been a part of for over 22 years. Without their support, camaraderie, esprit de corps, and core values, I would not be where I am today. It has been such an honor to be a part of the finest institution the world has to offer. To all Marines past, present, and future, OOH RAH and Semper Fidelis.

Without a doubt, I must thank all the celebrities I have worked with over the years for their dedication and belief in what we were doing together, even though it was VERY VERY TOUGH starting out. The end result was well worth it.

To my literary agents from my home town of Chicago—Jonathan Scott. Thank you for your tireless efforts and hard work. To the Rodale editors and the crew at the photo shoot for this book in Emmaus, PA (even though I never got the smile of approval from Joanna until we wrapped). In addition, a special thank you to Nancy Hancock at Rodale for her support, vision, and belief in this project.

Last but not least, a big OOH RAH and thank you to Christina Zaba and Roger Tavener of Prone for their skill and dedication in writing this book with me. They worked tirelessly in bringing the team together and I have appreciated working with them and have enjoyed their professionalism. It has been a great and long journey, but we finally did it. I cannot wait until the next one!

index

Boldface page references indicate photographs. Underscored references indicate boxed text.

F

U

Upper back stretch, 63, **63**, 95, **95**, 110, **110**, 153, **153**, 168, **168**, 209, **209**

V

Vegetables, 265, 266, 273, 280, 282

W

Walden, Harvey IV (author)
  Ask Harvey Web site, 9
  athletics, 273–74
  brother (Milton), 2, 269–74
  children (Tiyauna and Harvey V), 3–4, 21, 244–51, 272
  cooking by, 272–73, 275
  cousin (Randy), 271–72
  diet, 5–6, 262–67
  drill instructor, 2, 5, 11–12, 41–45, 147
  early years, 1–3, 269–74
  enlistment in Marine Corps, 1–2
  father, 2, 269–74
  godfather, 270–71
  grandfather, 254–56, 270
  grandmother, 265
  martial arts, 2–3, 254–56, 270
  meditation, 254–59
  mother, 269, 273
  motivators, 3–4, 243–51
  music choices, 123
  Officer Candidate School (OCS), 48
  retirement from Marine Corps, 251, 297
  statistics, 263
  television career, 6–8
  time management, 9
  uncle (Milton), 270
Walking, power, 20, 290
Waller, Rik (celebrity), 275
Warm-up
  calf stretch, 65, **65**, 112, **112**, 170, **170**
  chest stretch, 62, **62**, 109, **109**, 167, **167**
  groin stretch, 66, **66**, 113, **113**, 171, **171**
  hamstring stretch, 64, **64**, 111, **111**, 169, **169**
  low back stretch, 68, **68**, 115, **115**, 173, **173**
  march on the spot, 56, **56**, 103, **103**, 161
  neck stretch, 59, **59**, 106, **106**, 164, **164**
  quad stretch, 67, **67**, 114, **114**, 172, **172**
  shoulder stretch, 61, **61**, 108, **108**, 166, **166**
  side straddle hop, 58, **58**, 163, **163**
  side straddle hops, 105, **105**
  steam engines, 57, **57**, 104, **104**, 162, **162**
  triceps stretch, 60, **60**, 107, **107**, 165, **165**
  upper back stretch, 63, **63**, 110, **110**, 168, **168**
Water aerobics, 290
Water consumption, 263
Wheat bread, 264
Whole grains, 280
Wide push-ups, 77, 77, 180, **180–81**
  2 down, 2 up, 128, **128–29**, 188, **188–89**
Workout
  frequency, 28, 38
  journal, 31
    location, 35, 46
    music, 123
    time needed, 34

Y

Yogurt, 37, 264, 267

YOUR FREE 30 DAYS OF PERSONALIZED CELEBRITY TRAINING IS JUST ONE CLICK AWAY.

You've got zero excuses now. Get a 30-day <u>free</u> trial of Harvey Walden's no-excuses celebrity workout program and Ian K. Smith, M.D.'s, expert diet planning based on his *New York Times* bestseller *The Fat Smash Diet*.

What do you get? Try daily and weekly meal planners, customized progress charts, personalized exercise plans, recipes, and an online community. And a solid program to help get the weight off. Fast.

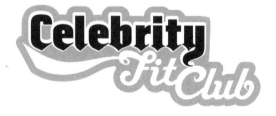

For your free 30-day trial, go to:

www.celebrityfitclub.com/noexcuses

Use this access code: A5Z37R